T0017090

Praise for *Decolonizing Wellness*

"*Decolonizing Wellness* holds no punches and I love it! Dalia does an amazing job of not only naming the toxicity that queer folks of color come up against in their wellness journey but also providing useful tips on how to make things work for you at your pace—while being patient and kind to your mind and spirit along the way. This book is a must-read for Black and brown folks who want to live their best lives, and a necessary tool for white allies that desire to open their lens and create positive spaces for people of all backgrounds."

—Nik Whitcomb, casting director and equity in theatre activist

"I have been hungry for a book to explore the intersections of self-care and body image before I had the language to truly understand what I wanted and needed. This book is a lifeline for the QTBIPOC community—particularly those who feel like they have been screaming from the margins just to be given the same amount of care and acknowledgment when it comes to holistic health. As a queer Asian woman, I am grateful that a resource like this exists. Dalia's compassionate honesty about the oppressive systems we live in—how that shapes the punitive and damaging diet culture we live in—is not only revolutionary but deeply needed for us as a society to heal both personally and collectively. If you identify as QTBIPOC, get this book now. And if you don't, you should still get this book now; it'll give you the deep understanding and perspective of how it feels to live in a marginalized body."

—Kim Thai, founder of GaneshSpace, Emmy Award–
winning producer, writer, and wellness advocate

"As a queer Black woman, I am so grateful that I finally have a wellness book that speaks directly to me. In this world, 99.9 percent of media is created for the white case—not this book. This book is important. This book is NECESSARY. This book illuminates why none of the other wellness books for 'everyone' felt like they could really work for me. There were so many times that I was reading this book and said "YES!" After reading this book, I feel like I have finally found the key to understanding why I've felt unwell, even after doing all the things that the diet and beauty industry have sold me. The world needs more books like *Decolonizing Wellness*. Dalia keeps it real about the external powers at play impacting my wellness as a person of color. (Finally, a book that doesn't shame my willpower or discipline for not being super skinny.) This is a book that I will read on repeat because it's full of incredible truths, wisdom, and exercises that I can return to for years to come. I'm so grateful that Dalia wrote this book for ME and other QTBIPOC+ folks like me. I felt so completely seen and understood by this book and as a queer Black woman, that feeling is rare. This book was a healing balm for my heart and soul."

—Gieselle Allen, mindset coach for women and femmes of color

"Health narratives for wellness oftentimes exclude circumstances specific to persons of color. Dalia Kinsey captures the essence of our wellness struggles and lovingly paves a way of escape for those trapped in marginalized ideas about beauty. *Decolonizing Wellness* is true to its name and a wonderful journey to self-acceptance and freedom."

—Dr. Dontá Morrison, activist and motivational speaker

"*Decolonizing Wellness* is an absolute must-read for anyone who wishes to truly maintain well-being and healing. Dalia's words are an authentic and important perspective of the harmful narrative that permeates the wellness industry. Dalia's critical yet compassionate voice is a much-needed presence that left me contemplative and validated."

—Felipe Gonzalez, yoga teacher

"As a Black, fat, queer, gender nonbinary person, I am constantly and consistently harmed by tools that are meant to help me. This is not the case with *Decolonizing Wellness*. Dalia has brought forth a text that bridges the physical, mental, emotional, and spiritual gap that people who live at multiple intersections tend to fall through when dealing with eating disorders. I can't wait to share this with my therapist and recommend this tool for other people struggling to nourish themselves in a world that seeks to destroy them. Thank you, Dalia, for this unique and sorely needed love offering."

— Rawiyah Tariq, witch, artist, healer, and speaker

"Never has a book encompassed what it is like to be a dietetics student or a clinician of color quite like this book. Dalia delivers with each chapter and page. *Decolonizing Wellness* truly opened my eyes and provided an intersectional approach to navigating the health and wellness space."

—Whitney Trotter, registered dietitian and RN, antiracism educator, and human trafficking activist

Decolonizing
Wellness

Decolonizing
Wellness

A QTBIPOC-Centered Guide to Escape the Diet Trap, Heal Your Self-Image, and Achieve Body Liberation

Dalia Kinsey, RD, LD

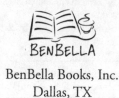

BenBella Books, Inc.
Dallas, TX

This book is for informational purposes only. It is not intended to serve as a substitute for professional medical advice. The author and publisher specifically disclaim any and all liability arising directly or indirectly from the use of any information contained in this book. A health-care professional should be consulted regarding your specific medical situation. Any production mentioned in this book does not imply endorsement of that product by the author or publisher.

Decolonizing Wellness copyright © 2022 by Dalia Kinsey

All rights reserved. No part of this book may be used or reproduced in any manner whatsoever without written permission of the publisher, except in the case of brief quotations embodied in critical articles or reviews.

BenBella Books, Inc.
10440 N. Central Expressway
Suite 800
Dallas, TX 75231
www.benbellabooks.com
Send feedback to feedback@benbellabooks.com

BenBella is a federally registered trademark

Printed in the United States of America
10 9 8 7 6 5 4 3 2 1

Library of Congress Control Number: 2021034774
ISBN 9781637740309 (trade paper)
ISBN 9781637740316 (ebook)

Editing by Vy Tran
Copyediting by Lyric Dodson
Proofreading by Doug Johnson and Laura Cherkas
Indexing by WordCo Indexing Services, Inc.
Text design and composition by PerfecType, Nashville, TN
Cover design by Kimberly Glyder
Cover image © Shutterstock / Rolau Elena; birds by Kimberly Glyder
Printed by Lake Book Manufacturing

Special discounts for bulk sales are available.
Please contact bulkorders@benbellabooks.com.

To my ancestors, known and unknown

CONTENTS

INTRODUCTION

Decolonizing Your Mind

Somewhere, on the edge of consciousness, there is what I call a mythical norm, which each one of us within our hearts knows "that is not me." In america, this norm is usually defined as white, thin, male, young, heterosexual, christian, and financially secure. It is with this mythical norm that the trappings of power reside within this society. Those of us who stand outside that power often identify one way in which we are different, and we assume that to be the primary cause of all oppression, forgetting other distortions around difference, some of which we ourselves may be practicing.

—Audre Lorde, "Age, Race, Class, and Sex,"
in *Sister Outsider: Essays and Speeches*

When I first applied to enter the nutrition program at Georgia State University, I was clear on a few things: I wanted to help underserved people improve their health outcomes and reduce their risk of preventable diseases

1

through dietary change and weight management. At the time, I was fully immersed in unscientific diet culture and hadn't started to investigate the role systems of oppression and entrenched power structures play in Western health promotion. I didn't question the lack of evidence to support the conflation of body weight and health status. After years of research and working with clients, I've come to understand that the stress of being marginalized is a much larger contributor to health disparities than are eating habits alone. The medical community's ongoing failure to feverishly address the chronic stress induced by institutionalized racism as a public health crisis is unconscionable. Evidence suggests that fighting inequity is a far more legitimate battle than fighting obesity in the name of defending the nation's health. It makes sense to question who stands to benefit from the propagation of weight bias and unchecked racism.

As my understanding of nutrition science grew, it became increasingly evident that the instruction dietitians were being given was heavily influenced by social bias. It is so easy to be blind to your areas of privilege. At the time of my program, I was young and thin. Initially, I didn't question the weight stigma that was evident throughout my studies, but after repeatedly hearing nonsensical explanations for health disparities, I started to question the validity of instructors' and researchers' assumptions. The assertion that ethnic minorities were to blame for health inequalities didn't sit well with me. The self-righteous ridicule of consumers for "ignorantly" clinging to cultural foods smacked of cultural centrism. It didn't seem realistic to believe that if people of color (POC) could just be convinced to eat in a uniform/assimilated way, they would magically enjoy all the same positive health outcomes of the dominant culture. You can't drink a green smoothie and cure the damage of unrelenting stress and the low-grade terror that comes with possibly being attacked, humiliated, or harmed at any moment for simply existing.

Bias needs to be controlled for in research. The goal of the scientific method is to protect against bias and uncover objective truths. As the majority of researchers are part of the dominant culture in the West, it makes sense to suspect that cultural centrism could compromise the objectivity of studies. There are several ways bias can creep into studies and distort conclusions, with one being that bias causes researchers to both ask the wrong questions and misinterpret data.[1] Yet it is no surprise that researchers surrounded by white supremacy in subtle and overt forms in their daily lives are minimally vigilant against racial bias. It is disappointing but not surprising that researchers chronically fail to be aware of their cultural assumptions. It is even less surprising that professors and educators fail to adopt cultural relativism and employ critical-thinking skills when examining the role institutionalized racism may play in health outcomes for marginalized groups.

At no point did my instructors acknowledge the horrendous track record of Western science in the realm of ethics and objectivity concerning race. My professors wholly ignored the possibility of ongoing weaknesses with cultural relativism compromising research. I don't recall a single encounter with someone who was open to the concept of looking at confounding factors that contribute to adverse health outcomes for people of color. My classmates were far more interested in hearing from white researchers than the people of color in the room. Whitesplaining and racial gaslighting were the hallmarks of my educational experience. Whenever I asserted that researchers were making logical leaps and that the study summaries were lazy combinations of conjecture and unquestioned bias, my peers countered with eye rolls and stony silence.

Whitesplaining: the act of a white person explaining topics to people of color, often in an obliviously condescending manner, and especially regarding race- or injustice-related issues.

Racial gaslighting: undermining the lived experience of others, shifting the focus from the racial injustice experienced by the recipient of abuse and their perceptions, triggering self-doubt, and discouraging victims of racism from speaking out.

Even though my voice was ignored on more than one occasion, photographs of me were repeatedly plastered on the department website. Using me as a prop and exploiting my skin color for the sake of marketing was a higher priority than making sure I was getting what I paid for: a comprehensive education where I felt welcomed rather than just tolerated. Unfortunately, there is nothing unique about my experience. Being silenced and simultaneously commodified or leveraged for the profit of institutions that claim to support us is a constant frustration for so many people of color.

The prevailing narrative is that you will be rewarded with acceptance and access if you are a "well-behaved" person of color. This is a lie. No matter how well I behaved, I could not access equal treatment during my time at university. This experience has echoed throughout my life and throughout the lives of other marginalized folks. Doing what white supremacy culture demands of us yields no protection. People of color are continually met with rejection and disrespect as we comply, even as we flout stereotypes and exceed expectations. A lack of economic access is not the problem; it is only a symptom. Systemic oppression is the disease. White supremacy, unchecked bias, and racism are the real reasons that less than 3 percent of registered dietitians in the United States are Black.[2]

After graduation, I was so burned out and demoralized that I questioned whether working in the field of nutrition was my path after all. I took a year-long break from nutrition to recover. Eventually, I recovered enough emotional energy to obtain my Registered Dietitian (RD) credential and accept a position related to my studies.

When I got my first job working in public health, I thought my initial goal to work with high-risk populations had come to fruition. During the honeymoon phase at this new job, I felt like the mission and work were perfectly aligned with what I wanted to do. Everything was going great—until it wasn't.

The longer I was there, the more the obsessive focus of the majority-white staff (and the exclusively white leadership) on weight and policing Black and brown bodies started to wear on my nerves. It became clear that we were not serving anyone by adding food preoccupation to the already-long list of things weighing on our clients' minds. The department obligated program nutritionists to weigh clients at every visit and "gently" remind them to strive for low BMIs. The mandatory weigh-in at all nutrition counseling appointments was beyond ineffective; it was harmful. Body shaming and body policing were only adding to the day-to-day stress of clients *and* employees. The individuals responsible for designing the programs were not connected to the people they were attempting to serve. They were clearly failing them.

Again, I started looking for research to explain why it felt like no real progress was being made toward health equity. I wanted to know what other explanation there might be for the health disparities I saw firsthand. I dove into women's studies, studying racial bias, weight stigma, fatphobia, and minority stress theory. I started to revisit many of the things I'd been taught at university with a more critical eye. I started reading research on my own without the biased filter of an instructor.

The standard rhetoric regarding personal responsibility for health-promoting behaviors is flawed. The role that racial and gender bias have played in how dietitians and other health professionals conflate fatness with health risk is powerful and often overlooked. Although there has been pushback against the dubious science that supports fatphobia and elevates some bodies over others in recent years, the body positivity movement has also become an environment where white- and hetero-centeredness often goes unchallenged. Take a look at the umpteen books on the market for the body-positive crowd; it's clear that some people think the universe is exclusively populated with white, thin-to-plump-sized, cisgendered women and their similarly complected opposite-gender partners. As a result of this incorrect assumption, the overwhelming majority of self-help books that deal with body image and food aren't equipped to serve as powerful wellness tools for people of color.

I doubt any of these writers had malicious intentions. Still, it is the default to view marginalized people as invisible when you are a part of the domineering cultural group. Avoiding the pitfalls of unconscious bias and minimizing the harm you do to others requires analysis and personal awareness. This is an ongoing process and hard work—work that a disturbingly small percentage of people are willing to do, preferring instead to remain wrapped in the comforting embrace of white supremacy delusion. Occasionally, I feel that progress is being made, but most resources fall terribly short of making people outside of the dominant culture feel welcome. It's rare to find content that resonates and doesn't seem tedious, overprivileged, and out of step with the reality many of us are living.

This book is the resource I was looking for. A guidebook written to nurture people of color and queer folks, centered on our unique lived experience. A book to spark a more in-depth intersectional conversation about body positivity.

MISS US WITH THE FAUX ALLYSHIP

People are starting to wake up to the fact that an overwhelming number of self-proclaimed allies have been complicit in silencing, diminishing, and, yes, oppressing their "friends" of color. These well-meaning folks often stop people from really being able to live a lower-stress, happy life by acting as though we live in a "post-racial" society because we had a Black president that one time. It's the same logic that allows many people to pretend that heterosexism has gone the way of the dinosaur since the US Supreme Court legalized same-sex marriage. The assertion that everything is fine when you know that things most certainly are *not fine* really does a number on your brain. Enter cognitive dissonance, the discomfort we feel when our actions don't match what we know to be true. It takes mental and emotional energy to behave as though everything's OK because you don't want to be accused of being oversensitive. Fear of further alienating yourself from the people around you, who make up the majority of the population and who don't share your marginalized identities, can make stuffing your feelings down and eating your words feel like the only option.

Suppressing your emotions is not a health-promoting behavior. Living with this level of fear and anxiety adds to baseline stress levels and undermines the body. The same people who claim to be so worried about health outcomes for Black and brown folks betray their insincerity when they fail to focus on the toll that living with racism, heterosexism, and cissexism has on us. Policing the behavior of marginalized folks under the guise of protecting them is a symptom of white supremacy, not a legitimate public health intervention.

I think it's obscene that we are ever asked to pay to consume media or resources that make us feel less than. It's one thing to happen across something that undermines your sense of self as you go about your daily living, but it is quite another to be asked to *pay* for that trash, then perform gratitude. I'm not here for the scraps.

Let me give you a real-life example. In the introduction of a book focused on body positivity, the author opened by acknowledging her unearned privilege as a white cisgendered straight woman. She posited that because she had no way of understanding the experience of people who don't look just like her and express gender in the same way as her, she should not even attempt to include any content for people who are not white, cis women. She then explained that that was a good thing: using her ignorance to opt out of lifting so much as a finger to create an inclusive resource was positive. Woke, even.

Ignorance is not an excuse for racism. Feigning ignorance or being willfully ignorant does not exempt individuals with privilege from a moral obligation to be actively antiracist and attempt to reduce harm perpetrated by systems of oppression. By the time you're reading that part of the book, you have most likely purchased it. Before you even get into the meat of the content, the author explains that she didn't create the resource with you in mind. While she is aware that you exist and understands that you probably picked up her book because you are in a state of suffering and need guidance that will help you take a few steps closer to loving and accepting yourself—too bad; you're the wrong color. The writer could not be bothered to do any kind of research that would make it possible to address any of the unique ways your body image has been affected by the dismissive treatment you receive in the world. Basically, you're just not important enough for the extra effort, but thanks for buying the book, and maybe if you dig through all this other stuff, you'll be able to find some crumbs that resonate with you.

If you have one marginalized identity or more, you are no stranger to consuming content that ignores your lived experience. While I certainly don't think every creation can or needs to be meant for all people, it is taxing to find yourself so rarely represented in the media you consume. Imagine that every time you search for nail color or hair color inspiration, you know beyond a shadow of a doubt that the first ten pages of Google results will not have a single representation of a person with your complexion. Imagine how annoying it becomes to see that manufacturers and advertisers continually accept your money and fail to offer you equal access to their products and services. The constant overlooking of people of color is evident even in first aid classes, where bruising is described only in terms of white skin. This marginalization can be fatal in cases of skin cancer,[3] and mortality rates for people of color with skin cancer are significantly higher than for their white counterparts.[4] Clinicians are often undertrained on how to care for people of color, making racial bias deadly in medical care settings.

When it comes to works focused on healing, the more something tries to appeal to everyone, the less likely it is to have the power to impact anyone significantly. That is why it is so vital to have content centered on frequently ignored identities. The beauty of our modern times is that, by and large, the gatekeepers to mass communication are gone. We no longer need permission to create content that resonates with people outside of the dominant cultural group. We no longer have to settle for scraps when it comes to the media we consume. There are creators who not only acknowledge our existence but celebrate our identities. These days, we all have the ability to make content that is specifically for our community. It doesn't have to be a major undertaking. Anytime you show up in the world as yourself, it's beautiful and it's healing for everyone who gets to watch. My social media feeds are a beautiful blend of lesbian and transmasculine thirst traps, humorous takes on shared cultural experiences of people of color, nonbinary humor, and trans queens dropping truth bombs. This book is my contribution to that growing body of work: a body acceptance–attuned eating guide for my beautiful rainbow-colored tribe that consciously rejects white supremacy, cissexism, and heterosexism but naturally continues to struggle with internalized oppression.

We are all complex, multilayered beings. Most of us belong to more than one affinity group. I hope to make you feel seen in the pages that follow, but I know it is nearly impossible to create something that makes everyone feel at home, so I want to acknowledge right here that I am not attempting to do that. This book is meant to speak to my fellow queer people of color who are rarely given anything that is made just for them. This book is the first of its kind, a body liberation book by a queer-identified registered dietitian of color specifically for queer Black, Indige-nous, and people of color (BIPOC) folks. I know how difficult it is to move through the world of self-help and personal evolution, attempting to become the best version of yourself without any resources tailored to your experience. I know how infuriating it is to realize that almost everything and everyone, even people you admire or resources you have found useful, finds you invisible or inconsequential. I know how hurtful it is to see self-help writers continually make resources without giving any thought to broad-ening their messaging to include folks who fall outside of the white, cis, het box. I know how maddening it is to watch fellow healthcare providers refuse to lift a finger to amplify the voices of providers of color who are uniquely qualified to share healing resources for other people with marginalized identities.

Identifying areas of disparity doesn't have to be soul-crushing. It is just information we can act on. We all have varying levels of access and privilege, but none of us are powerless. We can reject the treatments and social messaging that don't celebrate us and pursue what embraces us. Only when we can clearly identify our core values and desires and the blocks that society has put before us can we start to circumvent them and pursue our best lives regardless of the current state of affairs.

Reject the treatments and social messages that don't celebrate us and instead pursue what embraces us.

YOU DON'T HAVE TO BE STRONG

We have all heard the myth that Black folks are more resilient than other people. If you are a person of color, you have likely been praised by the dominant culture for powering through difficult situations without complaining. Through positive and negative reinforcement, we've been trained to act as though white feelings are more important than our lives, than our suffering. Rewards for stuffing your feelings down can come in subtle forms, but the consequences can ripple throughout your life. Something as simple as repeatedly praising a child for not bringing you any problems to guide them through can have damaging long-term effects. As we see women of color being celebrated by the dominant culture for overcoming adversity without any help or support, we can find ourselves slowly buying into the idea that we are superhuman: "Oh, Black women are just so strong." "We don't have the emotional or physical needs for care and safety that other people have." These are old lies created in support of white supremacy. Subjecting fellow humans to the atrocities of the transatlantic slave trade required logical leaps. It was convenient to believe that enslaved people did not experience pain as real humans/people of European descent did. The widespread nature of this lie continues to affect Black people in healthcare settings. In 2017, for example, Pearson drew negative press for reinforcing racist archetypes in medical textbooks.[5] Though the company vowed to revise the language in its textbooks and remove the racist assertion that Black patients do not require the same amount of painkillers as their white counterparts, this is a drop in the bucket. Racial bias, particularly anti-Blackness, has a strong history in Western medicine. Everything from unethical experimentation without consent to forced sterilization of Black Americans is just part of how that anti-Blackness has manifested itself in medicine. It is no wonder that many people of color are slow to trust healthcare services. In addition to the dominant cultural group's tarnished history with healing in communities of color, the dominant culture has largely dismissed traditional healing modalities. The consequences of these particular wounds of colonization are that people of color have been left disconnected from both their healing traditions and equal access to Western medicine.

The topics we will confront and the process of working through this book may feel heavy and difficult to take on. In the pursuit of true healing, discomfort cannot be avoided. This book is more than just a love letter to the baby queers and folks of color on their self-acceptance path. It is a plea for you to do the work it takes to learn to love yourself against all odds in a world that shows you so little of the love you deserve. It is possible to love and accept yourself in a way that goes beyond the superficial bod-pos one-liners you see major brands hijacking. No matter how unlikely it seems to you now, you can form a connection with yourself that is so strong and deep that it cannot be shaken. It is possible to know to your bones that you are worthy of peace, joy, and all the delicious things life has to offer.

As I'm writing this book, there are limited to zero resources giving voice to the experiences and issues around food, body image, and self-acceptance faced by marginalized groups and communities from the perspective of an actual member of those groups. Knowing what a disservice it is not to have a resource explicitly written with you in mind, *Decolonizing Wellness* is tailored to you, written through a lens and in a voice that you will find recognizable. You are too precious to be made to wade through scraps, sidestepping piles of microaggressions, casual racism, and heterosexism on your healing journey. You will not have to hodgepodge or cobble together something useful for your healing in the pages of this book. I know I have blind spots, just like everyone else. In this book's development, I reached out to other LGBTQIA+ folks, especially trans folks, for interviews and recommended resources to round out my perspective as a gender-queer, pansexual POC raised in an extremely religious household in the southern United States.

As a person with multiple marginalized identities, I am no stranger to society taking massive daily dumps on my self-esteem. It took years of therapy and personal growth to develop a genuinely loving relationship with myself. Getting to the point of not just accepting but celebrating each one of these identities took time. Incorporating triggers into my day that helped me revisit my goal of trusting myself and looking internally for validation and guidance was extremely helpful.

As I moved forward in my professional life and started working as a registered dietitian, it became more apparent to me how powerful using eating, an activity we engage in multiple times a day, every day, as a tool for untangling toxic internalized messaging could be. All things done repeatedly in life have the potential to be powerful affirmations. So many people have troubled relationships with food; it seems like an unlikely place to begin. But because of all of the drama and trauma that's wrapped up around body image and eating, trusting the body and learning to relate to the body and food in a positive way is an extremely powerful place to start. When you contemplate trying to undo years or decades of messaging, it seems so daunting. It can easily seem like an insurmountable task, too massive to know where to start. Feeding yourself is so tangible; it's a perfect entry point to create a major paradigm shift.

It's important to acknowledge that a lot of fear is likely to come up for us when we begin unraveling the negative messaging we have internalized about our marginalized identities.

Naturally, you may try to regain control or perceived control of the situation by jumping into overthinking instead of trusting the process. It is essential that you allow yourself to feel your feelings as you reconnect with your body and sit with discomfort. Because it is so easy to fool yourself into believing that you're making changes when in reality all you're doing is ruminating or thinking about making changes, you must focus on the action steps in the book. Instead of just intellectually processing the concepts we review here, allow each chapter to guide you toward action. The most important thing for you to do is take action. It doesn't have to be perfect. You don't have to know all of the steps you will take along the way. All you have to do is be willing to start. Commit to doing the work. The next steps will appear at the right time. The exercises and thought experiments in this book are meant to develop your sense of self-efficacy when it comes to nourishing and caring for yourself. We can't undo all of the trauma of stigmatization between now and the last page of this book. However, we can establish practices and an action plan to make healing and protective practices a regular part of your life.

This book's exercises are meant to help shield and protect you from the damage of both external and internalized oppression. Once you see the truth of the origins of body hatred, you will not be able to unsee it. Looking the truth in the face will trigger a paradigm shift in you that will make it easier for this book to fulfill its purpose of leading you to a greater love and greater appreciation for yourself. There is no wrong place to start. There is no wrong way to work through the process of improving your relationship with yourself and your body. The steps I present here in this book have worked for me and previous clients. If a step does not resonate with you, you can, of course, skip it. This entire process is about giving you what you need and supporting you and your growth, not burdening you with more "shoulds." Stay in a growth mindset as you move through this book and acknowledge that clarity follows action. All you have to do is be willing to start.

THE TRANSFORMATION AHEAD

Think for a moment about your absolute favorite friend. You love their quirks. You accept their flaws. They aren't always perfect, but your feelings for them never change. When you hear someone criticize them, you never, for a moment, agree or think less of them. Instead, you wonder how that person has completely misunderstood them. You effortlessly understand that if they don't love your bestie, it's about them, not about your friend, because after all, this friend is everything.

Now imagine what it would be like to have those same feelings and assumptions about yourself. At the end of this book, you will be closer to feeling that way about the person who looks back at you in the mirror.

Shame is so often our default, and guilt is an expected companion when facing our feelings of inadequacy or self-loathing. So before we embark on this journey of self-discovery, let's establish some ground rules.

1. Remember that shame, while natural, is not helpful. Whenever you feel yourself descending into a shame spiral, stop and acknowledge it. Talk or write it out; try to pinpoint what you are feeling ashamed about. Identifying the feeling and talking about it will reduce the intensity.

2. Be kind to yourself. The world can be a harsh place, but sadly most of us would be hard-pressed to find anyone who will beat us up as much as we do ourselves. There is no shortage of negativity and criticism in the world. Compassion, kindness, and understanding are all in short supply. Let's start to balance the scales by offering them to ourselves. Consciously make an effort to add to the amount of compassion in the world by starting with yourself.

3. Lean into uncomfortable feelings. When an emotion comes up for you, don't bolt. Ask this feeling what it is here to tell you. Develop a habit of processing your emotions so you can understand their purpose and release them—experiment with journaling and silent reflection. Scheduling time during the day to scan your body for physical indicators of stress and digging into where these feelings of discomfort originated is extremely powerful.

This book is dedicated to your healing and ongoing protection. We are going to take a look at our environment and how it attempts to do us harm. Recovery is a process. It took us years to internalize negative messaging. Decolonizing our relationship to our bodies and food will also take time. Use the spaces provided, including the extra blank pages at the back of the book, to complete the journaling exercises. Dedicate a supplemental journal as a companion to the book when you need additional space, keeping the journal next to your bed in the evening and on your person during the day so you can add notes when something comes up for you. Document proof that you are moving forward. While you don't have to do any of the exercises that don't resonate with you, I encourage you to question any resistance that comes up for you. Healing can be uncomfortable. Doing the exercises will create change if you give them time and attention. As you move through the book, notice which practices feel the most powerful. These will be the practices you will continue to revisit when you need to ground yourself.

We are going to learn how to shield ourselves. We are going to lean into love. We will use food to start a daily practice of self-affirmation and self-care that will take us further along the road to freedom and wholeness so the next time an internal or external voice implies we are unworthy, we won't believe it for a second.

RESPECTING YOURSELF
IN A HATEFUL WORLD

This was my first real big step toward self-degradation: when I endured all of that pain, literally burning my flesh to have it look like a white man's hair. I had joined that multitude of Negro men and women in America who are brainwashed into believing that the black people are "inferior"—and white people "superior"—that they will even violate and mutilate their God-created bodies to try to look "pretty" by white standards.

—Malcolm X, *The Autobiography of Malcolm X*

Where does internalized hatred come from? Naturally, it comes from living in a world that teaches us to hate ourselves. Everything and everyone around us contributes to our self-view—from the media we consumed growing up to the news and current events we follow, from our closest relatives and friends to our coworkers, caretakers, teachers, doctors, community leaders, and other individuals who float in and out of our lives. As a result of institutionalized oppression, we are surrounded by messaging that tells us we are not worthy of being seen, that we are "other than" the default majority and are somehow secondary. White supremacist, heterosupremacist, and cisnormative messaging is omnipresent. It is the air we breathe, and it's infectious. Quiet as it's kept, no one is exempt. Not only is it propagated by members of the dominant culture, but POC can exhibit white supremacist bias. Queer folks can and do bully and undermine LGBTQIA+ identities.

It is not uncommon for a person with one marginalized identity to adopt hateful supremacist views about other marginalized identities. A queer Black woman finds shelter and community within a group of Black folks and then is left out in the cold when heterosexism rears its ugly head. A transmasculine person finds connection and community with a local LGBTQ group and endures the slow reveal that gender-nonconforming people are not truly welcome in that space.

The damage that being othered does to our psyche is very real. Being bullied and stigmatized does not stop people from perpetuating harm and upholding the systems of oppression that disserve them. A common response to experiencing limited access to privilege is to scrap for status and relish opportunities to experience dominance over others, savoring privilege crumbs at every opportunity. The little-understood truth is that upholding systemic oppression is harmful, even to the people who seem to benefit from it.

We all experience varying degrees of privilege and stigmatization. Being on the receiving end of oppression is not a competition; there is no real benefit in comparing how much worse some marginalized identities have it than others, so we won't be participating in the Suffering Olympics today. Naturally, I am inclined to emphasize the damaging effects of anti-Blackness because of my lived experience as a Black American with Afro-Cuban and Jamaican ancestry, but the commonalities of the harm race-based trauma, minority stress, and micro-aggressions induce in regard to individual health is compelling. Humans are communal animals. When humans are stigmatized or ostracized from their immediate or broader community, it is psychologically damaging and, by extension, physiologically harmful. Whatever your marginalized identities, this is an experience you share with everyone who is othered by dominant white-cis-het culture.

THE ROOTS OF WHITE SUPREMACY DELUSION

No system or entity in the West has gone untouched by the damage of colonialism and the white supremacy culture it gave rise to. Our healthcare systems, religious belief systems, educational systems, governments, media institutions, beauty standards, and individual minds have all been tainted by white supremacy.

By the early nineteenth century, over half of the earth had been colonized by European powers. And because the dominant culture controls the narrative, the depth of harm that colonization caused has been largely glossed over in the Western world. Colonialism, even in antiquity, gave rise to racialized slavery, genocide, and ethnic divisions that still plague descendants of the colonized. The colonial era propagated the concept of scarcity and competition to many inherently collaborative and cooperative cultures, replacing the idea of strength as a community with

an obsessive focus on individualism. The ideology of isolation-
ism and individualism is uniquely that of colonization.

The world has suffered from accepting this ideology. Systems
of oppression easily stay in place and are unquestioned under
this framework. The concept of no one being free until everyone
is free is impossible to grasp through this lens, and the dominant
culture refuses to acknowledge the influence of bias and white
centrism on systems that purport to be objective, leaving many
practitioners incapable of offering healing or support to anyone
who is not a direct descendant of a colonizer and presenting as
such (read: white-presenting).

RACE AND HEALTH OUTCOMES

Modern science has revealed that there is no true biological definition of race. An incredible amount of genetic diversity exists
within racial groups, and a high number of genetic traits are
shared across racial lines.[1] Race is a social construct developed
and reinforced by the colonizer and spread worldwide to justify
crimes against humanity, including but not limited to robbing
enslaved people of their lives.

We all know that skin color, which is used as a main determi-
nant of someone's race, is real. But skin color is not inextricably
linked to any other biological trait.[2] Any feature you see in one
"race" you can find in another. For example, monolid eyes may be
common among people generally classified as Asian, but this eye
shape occurs in other racial groups. Moreover, it wouldn't make
sense to treat someone differently based upon their eye shape or
color. No one would believe you if you said that people with double lids were lazy, people with blue eyes were very athletic, and

people with close-set hazel eyes were more likely to be promiscuous. It is so clear that it makes no sense to draw these conclusions based on the features of someone's eyes. And yet, as a society, we continue to fall for the ridiculous assertion that one physical characteristic—the color of someone's skin—tells us something meaningful about their health outcomes and proclivities.

Even though race is not biologically real, the scientific community at large continues to operate as though it is.[3] Researchers continue to break people into these arbitrary unscientific groups. This tells you that the scientific process can be corrupted by the norms and beliefs of the day. There is a reason why "believe nothing you hear and half of what you see" is sage advice. Using critical-thinking skills and accepting nothing at face value is a vital skill for all people, but especially for marginalized folks. Remember that systems of oppression have the potential to affect how every single person operates.

Even though it's been established again and again that race is not scientifically real and that it's a social construct, people are genuinely surprised and confused whenever they hear this explained. While race is a figment of our collective human imagination, it absolutely affects how people's lives play out because society consistently upholds this belief system. The effect of marginalization and the consequences of being treated poorly because of racism are real. Not only are the consequences of racism real because of systemic changes that occur on a societal level in response to racism, the effects of racism are also real because simply believing that your racial or ethnic group has innate characteristics that are unfavorable changes the way your body and mind process information.[4] The experience of being racialized is real. It makes sense to acknowledge that the health disparities are real, but it does not make sense to believe that genetic predispositions are to blame for poor health outcomes. The logical conclusion is that these health outcomes are related to disparities in treatment.

Money and education don't serve as magical shields from the deleterious effects of racism. A Black person with a womb who has the same socioeconomic status and medical history as a white parent-to-be and who consistently accesses prenatal care may find no improvement in the likelihood that they will survive pregnancy. For example, Black women are three to four times more likely to die during or after delivery than their white peers.[5] When Black femmes express concerns about their symptoms, they are frequently ignored, delaying lifesaving treatment.[6] This is not surprising considering practitioners have been socialized in an environment that habitually disregards the voices of BIPOC. Racism is the ultimate preexisting condition; in fact, the impact of racial trauma on a cellular level is measurable.[7] Telomeres cap and protect the ends of chromosomes and are a fundamental part of cell division. As telomeres shorten in response to chronic stress, cell reproduction is compromised and tissues age. Telomere shortening over time is natural, but accelerated telomere shortening has been observed in marginalized individuals, contributing to increased risk for disease and shortened life expectancy.[8]

THE POVERTY SCAPEGOAT

Poverty is another favorite excuse the dominant culture often uses to blame marginalized people for their own suffering. If poverty leads to health disparities, then the story is that people should work harder to escape the cycle of generational poverty.

On the other hand, suppose systemic oppression is the cause of health disparities. In that case, all signs point to a deeper level of work needing to be done by the dominant social group. Who can monetize that? Why would a self-absorbed dominant cultural group want to do the work?

In contrast, "helping" people suffering from poor health outcomes brought on by chronic stress is very lucrative. Millions of dollars earmarked for minority health promotion are awarded to nonprofits every year. Simultaneously, minority-led nonprofits are consistently awarded less funding.[9] The dominant cultural group is able to make a profit off purporting to help marginalized individuals while shutting people out from actively creating their own solutions to health disparities affecting the communities to which they belong. As the dominant group shirks responsibility, they exempt themselves from blame and responsibility to change.

All too often, public health and medical communities use poverty as a scapegoat instead of addressing the fact that racism has compromised healthcare systems and individual practitioners, leading to higher death rates for Black patients regardless of income levels. It is undoubtedly true that because Black folks' ancestors were blocked from accumulating generational wealth, Black Americans are disproportionately vulnerable to economic insecurity. Yet time and time again, we've seen that money cannot protect us from racism. So, limited access to wealth and healthcare can explain some health disparities but certainly not all. When someone continually blames economics, they are also implying that if people just did better and were more successful financially, everything would be fine. That simply is not true. Money is not an impenetrable racism shield. Money certainly helps, but—news flash!—racism is a problem. Racism is a public health crisis.

RACE-BASED TRAUMA IS REAL

If you hold marginalized identities, you have been socialized to downplay and disassociate from the pain that stigma and marginalization cause you. As social creatures, humans find it incredibly painful to be excluded by others. It is human nature to want to belong. Early in human history, belonging meant the difference between life or death. When you are not allowed a seat at the table, when you are treated as invisible, it awakens a visceral fear.

Being othered throughout your life has taken a natural toll on your mental well-being. That stress, combined with the potential stress sensitivity as descendants of trauma survivors or from surviving adverse childhood experiences, makes many of us vulnerable to high levels of psychological distress and depressive or anxiety symptoms.[10] The mind is very resilient and very invested in your preservation. It will do what it must to protect you. Many reactions to chronic abuse may seem illogical or unhelpful when we look at them with a critical eye, but the brain and the body do what they have to do to survive. In an attempt to protect you from future harm, your brain and body may either develop a heightened sensitivity to threats of discrimination or they may resort to numbness. Race-based traumatic stress injuries can come from direct experiences of one-on-one racism, but they can also be triggered by witnessing racism. Symptoms of race-based traumatic stress can include depression, anger, headaches, chest pains, insomnia, and low self-esteem (more on this later). Suffering from race-based traumatic stress is not a mental illness in itself; it is a human reaction to prolonged stress exposure. Being subjected to race-based traumatic stress injuries does, however, increase your vulnerability to other mental health concerns,[11] especially if you have multiple marginalized identities.

MINORITY STRESS

Systemic oppression is a deadly preexisting condition. Psycho-social stress and minority stress theory summarize bodies of research that indicate that BIPOC and LGBTQIA+ individuals experience higher rates of poor health outcomes in response to the chronic stress of both institutional discrimination and perceived discrimination. While institutional discrimination blocks access to resources that support well-being (health care, housing, employment), the experience of interpersonal discrimination itself stresses the physical body and compromises overall health regardless of access to resources.

The expectation of rejection or attack compels us to be constantly vigilant. Being stuck in a hypervigilant stressful state for prolonged periods is at the root of minority stress. Same-sex couples that fear for their safety when holding hands in public suffer elevated stress during outdoor walks, even if nothing negative occurs during the walk. An Asian-American and Pacific Islander (AAPI) individual who continually witnesses anti-Asian violence on television experiences elevated stress related to their fear of racialized violence when they leave their home. A trans individual who is subjected to intrusive questioning from strangers about their genitals experiences elevated stress in social environments with new people who haven't established themselves as safe. A Black person being followed around a store while white shoppers are allowed to browse in peace is hit with a flood of stress hormones, as this seemingly minor insult serves as a reminder of the unrelenting disparities in treatment. A nonbinary person who receives employment paperwork requiring them to choose from two binary genders gets an anxiety-provoking reminder that the world is inhospitable to a key part of their being. All of these interactions are stress triggers. Minority stress is stacked upon the standard day-to-day stress the average person may experience.

When someone experiences stigmatization, discrimination, homophobia, and so on in their personal life, and observes others experiencing it as well, chronic stress responses are generated in the body.[12] If we look at the higher rates of depression, anxiety, and suicide among queer folks through a queer lens, it's pretty obvious that minority stress is to blame. The *Diagnostic and Statistical Manual of Mental Disorders* classified homosexuality as a mental illness until 1973. 1973! It is no wonder that bias in the mental health field still causes some practitioners and researchers to conflate queerness with a propensity for mental health disorders, pathologizing queerness itself. There is nothing wrong with our queerness. It is the hostility of the world around us in response to queerness that creates distress.

Anti-sodomy laws, for example, are a British import. In 1533, Henry VIII made it a crime for men to have sex with one another. When England was still hanging people for gay sex in the 1800s, there was an openly gay king in Uganda. In fact, prior to colonization, many Indigenous communities recognized gender diversity. Many Indigenous people of North America acknowledged the existence of a third or fourth gender, and *two spirit* is a Native American/First Nations umbrella term for transgender and gender-nonconforming folks. Ceremonial roles were often given to people who fell under this umbrella.

The concept of queer folks and trans folks being two-spirit people and hetero folks being one spirit existed in African nations as well. In precolonial Africa, there were far more open concepts of gender identity and sexual orientation. Tomb excavations have given us evidence of respected same-sex couples in ancient Egypt, and many deities were portrayed in a gender-fluid, nonbinary way.

Historically, the Igbo and Yoruba tribes of Nigeria did not have binary genders and didn't assign gender at birth. Instead, they allowed the child to grow and for the gender to reveal itself later in life. Other tribes were known to assign gender based not on physical genitalia but rather on the person's energy. Correlating gender identity with genitalia was introduced to many African countries by European colonizers.[13]

Gender variance is not new. We have always been here. Queerness and gender nonconformity are natural expressions of human diversity. Sexual orientation and gender expression are not phases people can be talked out of. People don't choose their orientation or gender any more than they choose their height or hair color. Treating people like trash for being themselves and living as who they know themselves to be isn't going to change natural inborn characteristics. Living in opposition to who you know yourself to be is incredibly harmful to your health. Suppressing your true identity can make you seriously ill. Prioritizing living your truth in the face of bigotry is a necessary act of self-preservation. Decolonizing ourselves and getting back to our roots logically includes removing homophobia and rigid binary gender concepts, along with internalized white supremacy, from our consciousness.

Learning to self-validate and overcome internalized stigmatization is extremely helpful in combating the damage of toxic messaging from the dominant culture. We are raised to believe that heterosexuality is the norm. Not having our identities reflected back to us early in life compounds the societal messaging that something is abnormal about our sexuality or gender presentation. Being devalued by your community and society at large leads to self-rejection, making it challenging for many of us to come out to ourselves, much less our loved ones. Crawling out from under the beliefs of heteronormativity and white supremacy delusion takes a tremendous amount of effort. White supremacy culture would have us believe that wealth is the cure-all for systemic oppression, focusing only on institutionalized discrimination. In reality, building community and spending time in affirming spaces is a far more powerful treatment for the damage systemic oppression does to the body. However, if we are struggling to reject the lies we've been told about our devalued identities, we will not be able to build healing relationships with others. The devastating truth is until we are able to heal our internalized stigma, we will not allow ourselves the opportunity to be seen and loved for who we are.

CONFRONTING SELF-HATRED

Let's look at some examples of how internalized stigmatization may present itself. You may see yourself or someone you know in some of these scenarios. This isn't meant to condemn anyone; it's meant only to raise our awareness of how we're socialized by the dominant culture to hate anything, even parts of ourselves, that deviates from what's considered the norm.

- A brown-skinned woman bleaches her skin.
- A gay man hides his orientation and openly condemns homosexuality.
- A trans woman avoids forming friendships with other trans people and is critical of how others present their gender.

- A Black American woman looks down on other Black American women for being too loud or culturally distinct.
- A ciswoman rejects forming relationships with other women, stating she would rather hang out with boys than girls because girls have so much drama.
- A second-generation immigrant cringes at the accent of the first-generation, non-native English speaker.
- A biracial woman straightens her hair and encourages others to do the same because it "looks more professional."
- A woman with monolid eyes gets plastic surgery to comply with a Eurocentric beauty standard that deems double-lidded eyes more attractive.

We are familiar with some, if not all, of these examples of internalized stigma, but what isn't always as clear is the damage that internalized oppression can have on our lives. Internalizing negative myths and stereotypes about the marginalized groups we belong to can lead to feelings of inherent unworthiness and buying into the belief that we are not capable, intelligent, or beautiful. Questioning our value and generally feeling unworthy often leads to low self-esteem, which affects how we show up in life and the decisions we make for ourselves. This is one reason some people are drawn to harmful processes, like skin bleaching, for example, which has become a global billion-dollar industry with no signs of slowing down.[14] The stronghold of colorism and European beauty standards are clear, as lightening creams and soaps are sold all over the world, reinforcing people's insecurities about their skin tone. Low self-esteem and negative self-image lead many to use these products, despite the expense and potential cost to their health when these poorly regulated formulas containing carcinogens, like mercury, are rubbed into the skin.

Beyond these tangible risks, low self-esteem has other insidious effects. Self-advocating, saying no to things we don't want, and pursuing our dreams are not possible if we doubt our value. When we don't have a positive self-image, we are left to rely on external experiences to figure out how to feel about ourselves. Negotiating condom usage and engaging in safer sex practices isn't feasible for someone who feels grateful to be seen. If someone is deeply uncomfortable with accepting compliments but finds themselves unquestioningly taking in negative feedback, they may have a wounded self-esteem. This is a very vulnerable, unstable position to be in. A poor sense of self motivates some people to work themselves to the bone, striving for external validation of their worth.

People-pleasing and putting the needs of others before our own to our detriment is a familiar symptom of a damaged self-esteem and poor conditioning to demonstrate our worth through service. The relief we get from outward markers of approval, like a romantic overture, a good grade, or an assessment at work, is only temporary. We crave a steady stream of positive reinforcement to counterbalance all of the negative thoughts in our heads. And if someone tells us we are a failure or too flawed to be loved, we are likely to believe it. A fractured self-esteem leads to feelings of helplessness, which breeds self-pity and indifferent default feelings. Looking repeatedly to others to guide or rescue us naturally interferes with our ability to be self-directed and live the lives we want.

Low self-esteem can also show up with a hard exterior. As a self-defense mechanism, some people become hostile and withdrawn to protect themselves from criticism that will confirm their fears that they aren't worthy. Someone seething with rage, who always goes out of their way to prove that other people's judgments don't hurt them, might not seem like they suffer from a damaged self-esteem. But going out of the way to break the rules and act as if the opinions of others doesn't matter is a cover. When our sense of self is fragile, isolating ourselves from others feels like our safest option.

In contrast, a healthy self-esteem offers stability because it is based on our clear understanding and acceptance of our innate value. When we understand that our worth is inherent, we are free to solve problems creatively and give up self-doubt and our desire for perfectionism. It's easier to make decisions that support us when we aren't constantly questioning ourselves. As our self-acceptance grows, we are able to resist comparing ourselves with others and are more likely to appreciate our unique traits. When our esteem is in a healthy place, we can stop underestimating our power, receive love, and value ourselves unconditionally.

The good news is there are several things we can do to turn up the volume on our positive thoughts. Although we can't expect to heal our self-esteem overnight, there are simple things we can do right now to start building our self-confidence muscles:

- Get away from people who tear you down. Seek out the company of people who hold up a mirror to your greatness.

- When someone identifies a positive trait about you, record it. Reference the list weekly and think of evidence that supports your positive traits. For example, if a friend says, "You have such a wonderful sense of style," don't dismiss or reject the compliment. If you feel extremely uncomfortable and all you can muster is a simple "Thank you," that is fine. But note this on your list. When you feel less charged and are in a neutral emotional space later in the day or week, think of examples that support the compliment. Your examples could be times when you felt fashionable or specific treasures in your home that your keen eye allowed you to spot.

- In addition to connecting with friends and chosen family who affirm you, intentionally select media that does the same. Even if the beat is amazing, if a song has homophobic messaging, it isn't worth listening to.

- Imagine what your life would look like if you knew you were worthy. What projects or passions might you pursue if you knew your self-worth wasn't at stake?

Despite our imperfections, everyone has value. It is human to be simultaneously flawed and beautiful. We are innately worthy.

RECOGNIZING SELF-ESTEEM WOUNDS

Low self-esteem can present itself in different ways, and they aren't always easy to recognize.[15] At the same time, not all people who suffer from discrimination and oppression turn this abuse inward. Allow yourself some quiet time to reflect on how you would honestly respond to these statements.

1. I feel crushed when someone criticizes my work or actions.
2. I feel like I deserve love and respect, no matter what I do.
3. After a failure, I feel immobilized.

4. People only respect me if I prove myself and keep up appearances.

5. I need to be liked by everyone I meet.

6. People only like me when I don't rock the boat.

7. If I am 100 percent myself, I will lose friends and social status.

8. I believe that someone who openly disagrees with me might still like and respect me.

9. I am afraid of being rejected by my friends.

10. I like myself.

If you agree with 1, 3, 4, 5, 6, 7, and 9, you might have internalized negative messaging that is undermining your self-esteem.

If you disagree with 2, 8, and 10, you might have internalized negative messaging that is undermining your self-esteem.

JOURNALING BREAK

How do you feel about your responses to the above questions? Do you feel uncomfortable? Where do you sense tension in your body? Are you experiencing feelings of shame or embarrassment? How can you be kind to yourself in this moment?

_____

_____

_____

_____

_____

Remember that we have all been steeped in white supremacy for years. We have the power to work against the toxic internalized messaging we find within ourselves, but we don't hold the blame for creating these toxic belief systems in the first place. When we accept that we have the power to change, we don't have to condemn ourselves for our previous behavior. Accept the beauty and power of our newfound reality; there are multiple ways to reduce the power hostile external forces have on our emotional and physical well-being.

CLOCKING EVERYDAY BIGOTRY

Microaggressions: brief and commonplace daily verbal, behavioral, or environmental indignities, whether intentional or unintentional, that communicate hostile, derogatory, or negative prejudicial slights and insults toward any group, particularly culturally marginalized groups.

You are able to read these words right now because your mind and body have been able to weather years of abuse. We might not think of microaggressions in terms of abuse, but what would you call it if someone was insulted every day for characteristics that are beyond their control but are central to their identity? The term *microaggressions* sounds as though these acts may be benign, merely annoyances. But being insulted and invalidated day after day after day for simply being yourself is anything but harmless. It has the power to break you down both mentally and physically.

Unfortunately, microaggressions are a part of daily life for many queer and BIPOC folks, and research is beginning to confirm that these small, everyday expressions of white-cis-het supremacy that are seen as benign have powerful health consequences.[16] One study established that after exposure to microaggressions, the study group experienced negative changes in their eating behaviors and increased anxiety, depression, and suicidal thoughts.

Microaggressions are often committed by people who consider themselves to be allies or who don't think themselves to be bigoted. Safe spaces are challenging to find. To escape microaggressions, you have to deliberately form community with like-minded folks where members make a conscious effort to keep their internalized oppression from spilling onto other people.

I know that if you give yourself the room, space, and quiet time to think about it, you can identify countless examples of someone who was supposed to be a safe person casually saying something that made you feel small under the guise of complimenting you. Let's try this exercise.

Set a timer for ten minutes. We don't want to spend a lot of time in this space. Write down every microaggression that pops into your head, everything someone has said to you that made you feel like crap. Whether it was someone devaluing your work and accusing you of being given something simply because of your color, because you couldn't possibly earn it on your own, or whether it was someone saying you're pretty for a trans woman or you're pretty for a Black girl, implying that people like you aren't usually pretty, that is a microaggression.

I completed this exercise myself and generated the following list in less than ten minutes:

- Accused of being offered a spot in the internship program because they needed a "Black girl"

- Told by a coworker that even though they didn't like Black people in general, they loved talking to me because "you aren't Black-Black; you are an Oreo"

- Congratulated for marrying a white person and *"mejorando la raza"* (improving the race) by an old friend

- Told by a stranger at an airport that they could tell I wasn't just a "regular Black" because I was too pretty

- Encouraged by other non-Black people of color to ignore a coworker who repeatedly used racial slurs to refer to clients (you already know which one) so I wouldn't be seen as difficult or angry by filing a complaint

- Advised by a close friend that I wouldn't be able to succeed in business if I focused on working with Black people because "you know they don't have any money; don't pigeonhole yourself"

- Asked how many children I have instead of if I have children (this one is constant)

- Told that I am paranoid and that racism doesn't affect me because I don't "live in the ghetto"

- Advised to avoid fried food and breaded meats (like fried chicken) during an appointment for plantar fasciitis while I was, in fact, a vegetarian, a dietitian, and not requesting weight loss advice of any kind

This trash is not harmless.

If, like me, you feel like it isn't fair that you have to deal with this type of treatment, you are right. It isn't fair. Dealing with microaggressions every time you leave the house is unfair and taxing. It isn't a moral failing to have trouble letting go of chronic abuse. Simply thinking positive thoughts will not erase the damage from daily insults. While the dominant culture may try to convince you that you should be grateful for all the progress that has been made, I encourage you to validate your feelings. To be fully processed, racial trauma must be validated. You don't have to be grateful for the abuse you receive. You don't have to be positive and upbeat about being kicked around. It isn't negative to acknowledge a fact. Now that you have identified some of the ways you have been harmed by systemic oppression in the form of microaggressions, let's take some time to feel your feelings and self-validate.

Look at the list of microaggressions you just created. Talk or write out the feelings they bring up for you and repeat this self-validation ten times, taking a deep breath between every repetition:

I have been wronged. I give myself permission to release this hurt.

See my examples below:

- When my academic and professional accomplishments were invalidated, it hurt. It was wrong that my coworker incorrectly assumed that I did not outperform my competition and earn my spot. It wasn't fair that my moment of celebration was tarnished by her insulting comment. I give myself permission to release the hurt she caused me.

- Being called an Oreo at work was a violation. Logically, I was hurt and offended to have my Black identity undermined. It's natural to feel hurt and betrayed when I realize someone who purported to be my friend is a racist. I give myself permission to release this pain.

- It's heartbreaking to realize that longtime friends are struggling with internalized white supremacy. Understandably, I was disappointed and heartbroken to hear a trusted friend use this incredibly problematic expression: "*Mejorando la raza.*" It makes sense that my old trauma around anti-Blackness among Latinx folks was aggravated by hearing this. I give myself permission to feel this heartbreak. I give myself permission to release my grip on this heartbreak.

- Backward compliments are tricky for me to manage since part of my socialization as someone assigned female at birth is to be gracious at all times. I forgive myself for not calling this stranger's compliment out for being backhanded and insulting. I did the best I could at the time. I give myself permission to release this pain.

- It is understandable that I felt betrayed and undermined when other people of color encouraged me to perform respectability politics instead of protecting my mental and emotional health in a hostile work environment. It is disappointing and heartbreaking when fellow people of color are ambivalent about anti-Blackness. I forgive myself for ignoring my gut and remaining silent. I forgive myself for letting fear of retaliation jeopardize my sense of personal peace.

- It is hurtful when people in my circle deny me support. I know it was natural to feel injured when my calling to serve POC was undermined by a "friend." I know it is safe to trust my intuition. I trust my higher self. I trust spirit. I do not need external validation, but I acknowledge that it hurts to be denied support. I give myself permission to release this pain.

- It is taxing to be burdened with the assumptions other people put on me. It makes sense that I am tired of explaining that I don't embody all stereotypes about Black people. I give myself permission to feel frustrated and angry that I lose time and energy to this on a regular basis. I give myself permission to feel my feelings. I also give myself permission to release the emotions that drain me. I don't have to hold on to this pain and frustration.

- Racial gaslighting is a form of psychological abuse.[17] I was justifiably frustrated and distraught when my lived experiences of racial injustice were dismissed. My feelings are valid. I give myself permission to release this pain.

- The compound stress of stigmatization because of race and body size is real. It isn't fair that when I visit a medical provider, my body size, race, and gender make it unlikely that my symptoms will be treated appropriately. I give myself permission to be angry. I give myself permission to advocate for myself. I give myself permission to release this pain.

Take your time with this portion of the exercise. Sit with any uncomfortable feelings that come up for you. What sensations do you feel in your body as you recall these experiences? How do these sensations change as you validate your feelings? Make a note of these shifts. You might be hit by intense waves of emotion. Lean into these. Your feelings are valid. Your emotions affect both your psychological well-being and your physical health. Honor your feelings and give them space.

When you are done, throw the list away. Give your body a good shake or dance to wring out some of the stressful vibes and return to the book.

START PROTECTING YOURSELF

It's important to be vigilant about what you allow yourself to be exposed to. It is time to become an expert at setting boundaries when well-meaning or not-so-well-meaning people do things to undermine your sense of self. This can take many forms, including people being willing to take your hard-earned money in exchange for substandard products or putting you on display for their financial gain in a disingenuous effort to perform inclusiveness. Under no circumstances should you participate in your own exploitation. Life is too short to exist in spaces where you are simply tolerated.

Appropriated oppression is something we can opt out of. It is something we have learned along the way, and it is something we can reject. Because we are working against years of consistent exposure to negative messaging, we need to be aggressive and strategic about our pushback. Learning to accept and approve of yourself is a stop on the road to freedom. Anything that undermines your ability to accept yourself is trash. As such, diet culture and weight stigma, which we'll discuss in the next chapter, are garbage you do not need in your life.

2

ESCAPING THE DIET TRAP

The scrutiny on our bodies distracts us from what's really going on here: control. The emphasis on our appearance distracts us from the real focus: power.

—Alok Vaid-Menon, *Beyond the Gender Binary*

Diet culture is the "system of beliefs that worships thinness and equates it to health and moral virtue, demonizes certain ways of eating while elevating others, pushes weight loss as a way to achieve higher status, and oppresses people who don't conform to the thin ideal."[1] Because diet culture is so deeply ingrained in our society and the pursuit of thinness has been erroneously linked to wellness without question for so long, most people require some convincing about dieting's health-eroding effects. After all, if it was so harmful, why would it be so widely accepted? You may think it almost has to be innocuous, as ever-present as it is.

Dieting is problematic on so many levels, I am only going to scratch the surface. There are a lot of resources out there (see page 147) that can help you deepen your understanding of why dieting is toxic and why you should have nothing to do with it, but in this chapter, I'll give you a few things to think about for now.

Reasons Why Dieting Should Be Avoided Like the Plague

- The thin ideal that is the motivational force behind dieting has racist and elitist roots.
- Dieting erodes self-image.
- Dieting takes up a lot of mental space and inhibits your ability to focus on things that are meaningful to you.
- Dieting drains pleasure from the eating experience.
- Dieting reinforces the idea that it is more important for you to be beheld or enjoyed by others as an object than it is to pursue things that bring you pleasure and satisfaction.
- Dieting is a powerful distraction from social justice issues.
- Dieting diminishes your sense of connection to your body and your ability to trust yourself.
- Dieting destroys autonomy and self-efficacy.
- Dieting leads to weight cycling and weight gain over time.
- Dieting is unhealthy, both psychologically and physiologically.

This list is not all-inclusive, but it gives us a solid foundation to work with. Let's flesh out some of these arguments a bit. Diet culture does not exist without the thin ideal at its foundation. This standard originated from the Eurocentric beauty aesthetics of the seventeenth century.[2] During the transatlantic slave trade, the desire to distinguish between the white perpetrators and beneficiaries of human trafficking and supposedly inferior enslaved people led to several pseudoscientific delineations between people of European and African descent. The cruelty and barbarism of enslaving other humans was so troublesome that both imagined and real differences were used to justify the crimes against humanity. Race science was used to identify traits of inferior and superior humans, leading to the bogus conclusions that Black people were lazy by nature and suffered from poor impulse control in relation to sexual pleasure and food, while morally superior people are able to resist carnal urges and maintain bodies that fit the thin ideal. Popularized in the 1800s, these racist claims continue to be popular signature tenets of anti-Blackness.

Dieting is a tool of oppression.

DON'T GET PLAYED

In her book *The Beauty Myth*, Naomi Wolf explains that dieting is a tool of oppression, a powerful distractor from meaningful things.[3] When we consider how much time assigned-female-at-birth (AFAB) women spend attempting to control their bodies and what percentage of their disposable income they spend on the pursuit of the ever-elusive beauty standard, it is nauseating.

When we think of how rampant misogyny perpetuates wage inequality and gender-based violence, it really makes us question what we are doing when we're spending this much money supporting companies that continue to distract women from more critical issues, like their own oppression.

"Your only value is physical beauty" is a lie that tends to affect femme-identifying people more than others, but the effect is definitely extending to other gender identities as companies decide to exploit other people's vulnerable sense of self for profit. Why are we bankrolling organizations that don't support our full liberation? How can we go from one fad diet to another and not wonder who we are really doing it for? Is this really something we want to do for ourselves or something we feel compelled to do, something we think we have to do because we have been brainwashed into believing that it's more important to be seen than anything else? Again, do we really want to participate in our own exploitation? Do we really want to play a game that was originally set up to oppress people of color and femme-identifying people? Do we really want to adhere to the beauty standard at all?

Let's take this just a little deeper. What is the motivating factor behind wanting to meet this standard? Could it be that our fear of loss of access to potential romantic partners keeps us stuck in this preoccupation with the beauty ideal? Have we made a subconscious connection between the pursuit of thinness and the pursuit of worthiness? Could it be we have created a community around the pursuit of the beauty ideal and are reluctant to let it go? Does a smaller body more closely fit the aesthetic norms associated with the gender we seek to be clearly recognized as belonging to?

DIET CULTURE AND THE BINARY

Femme folks are certainly not the only people suffering from body dissatisfaction and being preyed on by the diet industry. Cis gay men typically rank just under cis women in body dissatisfaction surveys.[4] There is an overwhelming emphasis on the body in gay male settings, and this body hierarchy is clear on dating apps. Apps allow you to filter by ethnicity and reductionist gay male body types, like twinks, otters, foxes, bears, etc. Users hide behind the word *preference* to validate being fatphobic, femmephobic, transphobic, racist, and ableist.

The tendency to associate muscularity with masculinity fuels gay gym culture. Exercising to the point of exhaustion or injury and severely restricting calories with the help of diet drugs is the norm for many. People who opt out of beating their body into submission are often ridiculed or body-shamed online. Higher rates of body dissatisfaction leave gay men far more likely to develop eating disorders than heterosexual men.[5] Mainstream queer and het adult entertainment also continually present lean, muscular, able-bodied cis men of tall stature as the masc ideal. Cis gay men and nonbinary masc folks who don't fit that ideal are left to reconcile what masculinity means for them if they don't fit that limiting standard. It is difficult to accept our individual bodies when we rarely see a variety of body sizes and gender presentations in a positive or neutral light.

"The image of a nonbinary person, now that we're starting to get some sort of representation, a lot of the times is limited to a white, very thin, masculine person, and that's not the reality for so many people," says Lashan, a Black nonbinary health educator. "You have to figure out what makes you feel most comfortable within yourself outside of white ideals."

The Western world presents us with such limited examples of gender variance that we easily get boxed in by rigid binary rules about gender. Dominant cis-het cultural messaging about body image influences us as much as anyone else. Because of this, transmasculine folks often find themselves drawn to restricted eating to induce weight loss and suppress gendered features to read more masculine in a binary way. Young trans and gender-nonconforming people are particularly vulnerable to eating disorders,[6] as they navigate living in a rapidly changing body with limited access to tools that support their gender identity. Hormone blockers, hormone therapy, gender-affirming surgery, packers, binders, tucking, breast prosthetics, and releasing rigid gendered body expectations that don't allow for body size diversity are all tools that can be used to address some of the things we are reaching for when we restrict eating in an effort to treat our gender dysphoria. When we are not able to access the tools that support our gender expression, the idea of exerting control over the body through restriction becomes very enticing.

The desire to be recognized as our true gender is so intense because it connects to the universal human desire to be seen and accepted as we are. We all work to avoid the pain of rejection. We naturally gravitate toward the limited tools we have access to, including the mainstream coding of fashion (skirts are for women, ties are for men) to communicate our gender identity to the rest of the world. In transphobic environments, not reading as cis carries with it not only the risk of rejection and verbal ridicule but physical danger as well. It only makes sense that many of us who aren't binary trans folks still expend massive amounts of emotional and material resources on performing gender in ways that we know the world around us will be more likely to accept. Passing is a complicated topic. It is understandable that many rely on passing for safety and survival reasons. Others see passing as an act of assimilation that holds no appeal. In the end, you have to decide what is right for you at this stage of your life.

Gender dysphoria: distress that occurs in people whose gender identity differs from their sex assigned at birth

Gender euphoria: an intense feeling of joy experienced when one's internal gender identity matches their external reality

If this resonates with you, don't judge yourself harshly for having a natural human desire to belong and seek approval from and connection with others. As a genderqueer nonbinary person, I continue to work through my desire to not be mistaken for a cis-woman without feeling forced to perform a narrow understanding of what it means to be nonbinary. For example, I am not thin. The very words we use to describe large bodies are feminized. The conflation between thinness and genderlessness is a limiting cage. Gender diversity occurs right alongside body diversity. It can be hard to know how to present ourselves when we have seen such limited representations of gender in the world around us.

Many people are still under the assumption that you can determine someone's gender simply by looking at them. Because society frequently deems menswear as gender neutral, AFAB nonbinary folks drawn to menswear are more likely to be believed when they present their nonbinary identity to others. However, if you are a nonbinary AFAB person who loves wearing dresses, you will be confronted with other people's limited ideas about what a nonbinary person looks like. The truth is there's no wrong way to express your gender identity. The rigid binary and the clothing we associate with it are heteronormative cages we don't have to continue being confined by. Your happiness is the only barometer you need to determine what is best for you. If binary gender expression lights you up, then that is what is right for you. Gender euphoria is the goal, and getting there requires abandoning your attachment to external approval and prioritizing your desires. Trust your intuition and follow your heart.

Suppose you are a ciswoman who feels best in traditionally masculine clothing. Wear that. If you are a femme-identified gender-nonconforming person and you feel like you are living your best life when your adornment isn't strictly hyper-femme, then do you. Of course, if popular binary femme trends appeal to you and spending your disposable income on beauty gives you life, then that is what you should do. I just encourage you to check in periodically and make sure that where you send your dollars continues to serve and resonate with you. It really is a matter of questioning why we are doing what we're doing and whether it is in service of the self. We have nothing to prove. Our bodies are our own. When deciding how to adorn our bodies, pleasing ourselves should be our primary concern. Prioritizing your happiness supports your health and the well-being of your entire community. The happier you are, the more health and happiness you'll be able to spread out or share with others. Happy people are more productive and creative and have more emotional space to help those around them.

Heteronormative and white supremacist standards of beauty aren't the universal ideals they present themselves to be. Nothing is more important than feeling comfortable in your skin. How you present yourself to the world is something only you have the right to decide. And you are always free to change your mind. True liberation doesn't aim to simply replace old shackles with new ones.

RECLAIMING OUR BODIES

Would you rather maintain a thin beauty ideal established by people who believed your ancestors were subhuman, or would you rather learn to feed yourself in a way that feels nourishing to your soul? Would you rather allow your body to be commodified and used to generate profit for people who care nothing about you, or would you rather learn to understand that your body is a connection to spirit, purpose, and all the people who came before you?

Giving up dieting requires that we let go of not only limiting beliefs about beauty standards and body hierarchies but also years of conditioning that lead us to believe we need external help to know how to live.

The body functions best when it's allowed to self-regulate. However, the oversimplified way we have been trained to understand food and body size makes trusting the body feel counterintuitive. The moralization of fatness and eating habits green-lights disrespecting people in larger bodies and creates a fear of fatness in all of us—and if you are terrified of fatness, you will recoil at the thought of allowing your body to lead you. Fatphobia will make you cling to the concept of manipulating body size through food and physical activity. Escaping the diet trap will require both a revaluation of our beliefs around body size and the trustworthiness of the body itself. Confronting the internal barriers we have to releasing dieting, honoring our appetite and cravings, and eating on demand is fundamental.

An imperialistic worldview pits humankind against nature. Naturally, populations that were subjected to imperialism and colonization continue to be suspicious of nature and the body by extension. The idea that there is a right and a wrong way to do everything is a very colonized, dichotomous way of seeing the world; if you view life in a holistic way, you'd have less trouble understanding that it is rare that anything is 100 percent negative or 100 percent positive. Everything is nuanced. Wellness is multifactorial.

We can't "green smoothie" away the damage of systemic racism and homophobia. Using fatness as a scapegoat eliminates culpability for people in positions of power who continually uphold systems of oppression. The dominant culture propagates the belief that the "obesity crisis" is to blame for health disparities in communities of color because BIPOC folks, unfortunately, are just so impoverished they don't have access to quality food. Or they're just so hopelessly not white that they struggle to fully adopt Whole Foods as the solution to all their problems. If only we could just educate them on our superior white eating habits, they would instantly experience longer life expectancies and better health outcomes like us.

The assertion is that ignorance keeps BIPOC in this loop of poor health outcomes. The obsessive focus on policing the size of Black and brown bodies in lieu of calling the dominant culture to task for terrorizing, suppressing, and bullying folks of color is reflective of the misguided assumption that white culture is ideal. Assimilation is the magic bullet. Being distinct from the dominant culture is problematic, not the abusive behavior of the dominant culture. How misguided! How can people operating under this assumption offer any true healing solution to folks of color? It is impossible to be a profound aide to anyone you hold in low esteem.

When you pile on the assumption that all fat people are to blame for being in larger bodies and for any health problems they may experience, tragically ineffective health care is what we get. Fat folks, folks of color, and queer folks are more likely to die from manageable conditions because of unchecked bias and low-quality care from providers. Another consequence of these unchecked assumptions for trans folks of size seeking gender-affirming surgeries is dismissive care and being blocked from lifesaving procedures because of BMI, regardless of other positive indicators of readiness for surgery.

As we discussed in chapter 1, racism explains health disparities far better than lifestyle factors do. Blaming the consumer or the individual for their habits is suspiciously convenient. It allows members of the dominant culture in positions of power to continue to believe that their norms are superior to those of minority cultures. And it enables them to occupy the ever-popular white savior position, where they're helping to civilize people of color for their own good. And oh, aren't we lucky that they're ready to help us?

But if you take a closer look, you will notice that the overwhelming majority of the people purporting to be so concerned about the health outcomes of people of color are complicit in the ongoing oppression of BIPOC folks. If you refuse to acknowledge that systemic racism is real, if you refuse to recognize that racism is affecting the health of your patients, then you are complicit in upholding systems of oppression—the same systems of oppression that are making people ill and multiplying people's risk of suicide, anxiety, and depression.

The amount of research available on the health consequences of chronic stress stemming from systemic oppression is obviously going to be limited. Studies and research aren't free. There has to be some economic benefit to performing the study for most research to be done. For some, the pursuit of knowledge is enough of a motivator, but the issue of funding is a barrier. The scientific community is frequently compromised because of funding sources. The absence of research on a topic that concerns you as an underrepresented person doesn't mean the problem doesn't exist. It could simply mean that the motivation or the economic incentive for doing the research doesn't exist. Western culture (and, by extension, all nations affected by colonialism) is money-driven. If there isn't a monetary reason to do something, you will be hard-pressed to get it done. It's not impossible, but the effort required to spearhead research that doesn't stand to pad someone's pockets is a hard sell.

The economic incentive to pathologize obesity is massive. Treating being in a larger body as a disease rather than accepting body diversity as a natural part of the human experience generates approximately $70 billion in the United States alone.[7] If you believe the weight loss industry is invested in the health of its customers more than profits, you are playing yourself. Whether your interaction with the weight loss industry is in the form of a weight loss program at a local gym or a medical weight loss intervention at your doctor's office, the program exists to generate income. Indications that dieting actually harms clients or patients are logically ignored when the sole reason for existing is to generate profit. It *is* possible to sidestep the damaging time suck that is dieting and focus on health-promoting behaviors, like finding movement you enjoy and eating in response to what your body signals, but how do you monetize that? Can you make billions of dollars telling people to trust their bodies? Predatory marketing that undermines individual confidence and convinces the consumer that they need to be fixed has a long and successful track record. Empowering consumers to purchase only what they need might potentially generate a sustainable income for individual coaches, but it won't ever generate billions of dollars.

So even though there isn't an abundance of research to reference, let's not undervalue our lived experiences. We can't depend on the dominant culture to validate what we already know. We don't have to find an external resource to back us up. In this warped system, we don't have time to wait for the majority to catch up to what we know to be true. I believe you. Your people believe you. You don't have to prove a thing in this space.

JOURNALING BREAK

Let's look at your personal history with dieting. When you answer these questions, consider both your personal diet history and what you have observed in friends and loved ones.

Can you remember a time when you ate whenever you were hungry without worry?

_____

_____

_____

_____

When were you introduced to the concept of "good" and "bad" or "healthy" and "unhealthy" foods?

_____

_____

_____

_____

Have you ever restricted certain food types outside of a formal diet?

_____

_____

_____

_____

Do you remember a time when you used your body to explore the world around you but didn't think much about its aesthetic appeal?

_____

_____

_____

_____

How did you feel about your body at the start of your first formal diet?

_____

_____

_____

_____

How did you relate to your appetite before dieting?

_____

_____

_____

_____

How did you feel about your body at the end of your first diet?

_____

_____

_____

_____

Describe your relationship to your appetite after your first diet.

_____

_____

_____

_____

On average, how much time and mental energy did food preoccupation and maintaining the diet take up for you daily?

_____

_____

_____

_____

Have you ever experienced weight cycling (rebound weight gain after dieting)?

_____

_____

_____

_____

How did you feel about your body after regaining weight in comparison to before the diet?

_____

_____

_____

_____

Has dieting ever made you feel good about yourself? If so, describe how long this feeling lasted and what followed.

_____

_____

_____

_____

Has dieting ever made you feel more comfortable in your body? If so, describe how long this feeling lasted.

_____

_____

_____

_____

There is no proven effective intervention for long-term weight loss. This is not to say that there are not anecdotal stories of people losing weight and keeping it off. What I mean is there is no *scientifically* proven intervention for *significant* long-term weight loss.[8] Long-term weight loss requires long-term effort. All the time and energy spent on dubiously healthful weight maintenance is not sustainable for most people. Literally, all interventions you have heard touted as foolproof have failed to prove themselves. When diets are subjected to scrutiny, they all fail to demonstrate a significant rate of long-term success.

The body is very resilient, and part of its resilience involves a relentless drive for homeostasis. Your body's primary focus is survival. Fat is not inert. Fat is metabolically active, and it works with the rest of your body to protect you.[9] Your fat does not care about arbitrary beauty standards. Your fat cares about survival. When your fat notices a decrease in the number of fat cells or a reduction in fat cells' size, it does all it can to send signals to the brain to stimulate your appetite and slow your metabolism to help you get back up to your previous level of body fat. Your body does not see an abundance of energy stores (a.k.a. fat) as a problem. Your body sees it as a buffer, potential protection from famine or periods of lack in the future. Since fat has protective work to do, the body is not inclined to release it. When your weight drops in response to restrictive dieting, your body pulls out all the stops to replenish your fat stores. In contrast, one of the best things you can do for your body to stop it from continuously storing excess energy is to show your body that it is safe, that it will be fed consistently, that when it sends a signal for food, it will be answered.

To date, the search for tools to fight the mechanisms the body has at its disposal to keep you at a steady weight has been fruitless. No one has found a tool powerful enough to prevent rebound weight gain. When you force the body to lose weight, it pushes back, and it pushes back hard. Most people end up gaining all the weight they lost and then some. As the body pushes a dieter to eat more, it turns up its own ability to hang on to fat, no matter how few calories one eats (through regulating metabolic rate) and how much one exercises.

Weight *gain* is the proven long-term result of dieting.[10] There's far more evidence to indicate that dieting can hurt you than there is evidence suggesting that dieting can help you. Considering the high failure rate of diets and clear connection with weight cycling, recommending dieting as a health-promoting behavior is unconscionable.

Remember to question everything. Who stands to benefit from pathologizing bodyweight diversity? Who is bankrolling the research? If that company or organization also wants to sell you something that just so happens to be related to weight management, don't ignore that clear conflict of interest.

WEIGHT STIGMA HURTS EVERYONE

Marginalized folks are being subjected to daily abuse. Fatness has been used as a scapegoat and an additional excuse for the dominant culture to opt out of accepting responsibility for increasing marginalized people's baseline stress levels. It's a natural human tendency to self-regulate emotions, to try to compensate for the damage of external stress through coping mechanisms. Some people's coping mechanisms involve restricted substances. Some people's coping tools are food or alcohol. Eating in response to stress is a common human coping mechanism. If you have noticed that you frequently use food to self-soothe, you are not a food addict. Binge eating in response to stress is the symptom, not the disease. The disease is systemic oppression. Systemic oppression is compromising the health of millions of people. Continually focusing on a natural reaction to chronic stress and demonizing fatness is not helpful. It creates obstacles to equal health care for people in larger bodies and encourages fatphobia and food obsession in thin people. The pervasive hostility toward fatness, deeming it an unattractive moral failing, is harmful. It is based more on learned bias than on scientific evidence.

Many of the adverse health outcomes that are continually linked to obesity haven't been proved to have a cause-and-effect relationship with obesity. Being in a larger body is not a death sentence. There is a difference between correlation and causation. Correlation simply means that when you observe one thing, you often observe another thing. Causation is cause and effect.

Suppose, for example, someone was to tell you that many cancer patients have yellow teeth and discolored nails, and based on that correlation, we decide to start cautioning the public against all the dangers of having yellow teeth and discolored nails. So, we work diligently on creating public health campaigns to warn people of the risks and educate them on all the simple changes they can make to protect themselves. Make sure you use a clear coat of nail polish before applying tinted lacquer to prevent discoloration. Protect your teeth from discoloration. Avoid drinking red wine and coffee.

Do you think these interventions will protect at-risk individuals from cancer? We know smoking also discolors teeth and nails. Will bleaching your teeth and continuing to smoke improve your risk? Will any of these warnings related to an observed symptom reduce the risk of lung cancer in smokers? Obviously not.

When we focus on weight as a gold standard to measure health, we are making a similar mistake. Yes, a lot of people in larger bodies also have health problems. Do we know that weight is the sole cause of these health problems? Could other factors be at play? Many poor health outcomes that are typically blamed on obesity could also be explained in part by the fact that people in larger bodies are denied equal access to health care. Higher body weight can also be a symptom of inadequate access to time and resources for self-care. If you are already in a marginalized group and you have been using food as a coping mechanism to manage your stress in response to all the abuse you get from the world at large, do you think having to deal with weight stigma in addition to your other external stressors is health-promoting?

When people pile on and further stigmatize your body, it does damage. A natural reaction to discrimination and fat-shaming is to disconnect even more from our bodies and eat for reasons aside from physiological hunger. The truth is, fat-shaming doesn't help anyone. Criticizing friends, family, or ourselves for weight gain, stigmatizing fatness, and insinuating that some bodies are unacceptable is destructive and not helpful on any level. Weight stigma damages health. Racism damages health. Colorism damages health. Homophobia damages health. Transphobia damages health.

Stigmatizing people is always destructive.

JOURNALING BREAK

A major protective step you can take to begin unraveling the toxic beliefs you have internalized about your body is to curate the media you take in. Let's start with a journaling exercise. Think of all the ways you have received negative or limiting messaging about your body and personhood. Make a list.

Include everything that comes to mind from parents, family members, friends, church, advertising, social media, the limited portrayals of masc and femme desirability in porn, TV shows you watched growing up, the magazines your mom used to buy, the songs you grew up listening to, and the disk jockeys who used to play them. Give yourself as much time as you need to write down everything that readily comes to mind, including old and current toxic messaging.

_____

_____

_____

_____

_____

_____

_____

When you are done, look it over. What can you completely cut out of your life? What can you edit? It isn't the eighties anymore. You can and should curate what you see. Shield yourself from anything you can identify as harmful to your sense of self. Limit your exposure to content that doesn't validate your lived experience or acknowledge you as part of the audience.

Super white, heteronormative shows that reduce people of color and queer folks to props with no storyline of their own are diminishing. It doesn't matter if there is no explicitly anti-gay messaging in the show. The absence of representation in itself is damaging. Similarly, the lack of body diversity on TV shows and in films impacts our ability to accept bodies of different sizes. Notice how fatness is framed when it is presented in the shows you watch. Is weight gain tragic? Is the fat character a hopelessly single sidekick, obligated to be a jovial, self-diminishing caretaker for the thin main characters? Look at your Instagram feed. Are the only folks of size on your feed plus-size models with flat stomachs and hourglass figures? Is it full of limited ableist, thin, white, and heteronormative representations of beauty? Of course, thin, cis white men and women can be beautiful, but so can everyone else. Being exclusively exposed to thin, cis white beauty as a gold standard is what is damaging. Curating a more inclusive feed will be helpful, but after a lifetime of seeing only one representation of beauty, it wouldn't hurt to give thin-white-cis-het-centered content a total break. Decolonize your social media feed. Grace yourself with a more diverse view of the human experience by filling your feed with people of different ages, body sizes, levels of physical ability, cultural backgrounds, and gender expressions. Queering and un-whitewashing your media is a crucial step in accepting that there are many ways to show up in a human body, and all of these forms are beautiful and quite all right.

FOOD AS A GROUNDING TOOL

There is far more that goes into living a healthy life than what you put in your mouth. Focusing on weight is not health-promoting. Striving for thinness at all costs has destroyed the health of countless individuals. Continually focusing on body weight in a negative way increases stress and internalized shame. That isn't healthy. So much of the obsessive focus we see with prioritizing thinness seems connected to the delusion that if you just eat the right things, you will live forever. That isn't how that works. As we look at shifting our view of what is important in terms of how we relate to our bodies and food, it's crucial to face the fact that our lives are finite. Our goal is not immortality through kale smoothies and carrot juice. We are here to live full, joyful, authentic lives. Any practice that we decide to take into our lives needs to be in alignment with that purpose. Instead of living under the delusion that we can achieve immortality through "good behavior," it is far more empowering to focus on treasuring the lives we have. It's important to live in a way that honors and celebrates the present as the only thing we have. It's important to make sure we are not compromising our purpose in an effort to pursue things that ultimately have no meaning.

Food can be used to help us stay in alignment. Food can be used to help us recall our divine nature. Food can be used to help us remember, in the thick of tumultuous times, that we are primed for survival. Mealtimes can be used to remind us that our personal judgment can be trusted. Information coming from our body at all times is pointing us in the right direction. Instead of food preoccupation being a distraction from the beauty of our brief time on this planet, we can use food to ground us.

Food is a great place to start developing our capacity to understand our needs and practice self-care in a way that mitigates the damage of a hostile living environment. Food is not a cure for everything that ails us, but it is powerful medicine when used to amplify the body's natural power to support ourselves, as a tool for self-care, free from shame and restriction. Food and movement can and should bring us joy, not stress. Anything we do several times a day can be an affirmation. We can use mealtimes to speak self-belief and self-acceptance into our lives.

Even though deliberate weight management is a lost cause, supporting overall health with a high-nutrient diet is not. The pursuit of thinness (or just the right amount of thickness) is *not* the only reason to eat food that nourishes and strengthens you. Eating a diet high in fruits and vegetables, full of high-nutrient foods, and finding forms of movement that light you up definitely support health. But eating a well-rounded diet rich in nutrients may or may not result in weight loss. If you have been trained to equate thinness to health, beauty, or worthiness, this realization can be devastating. The good news is you can work on purging those false beliefs from your mind. You can access health without compromising your self-esteem or sense of self. You don't have to be dependent on external cues for how to behave. Your body does not need to be tamed. Your body's ancient wisdom is the key to escaping the diet trap and realizing your own power.

EATING AS SELF-CARE

*Caring for myself is not self-indulgence, it is self-preservation,
and that is an act of political warfare.*

—Audre Lorde

We all have coping strategies for stress. The question is whether or not the strategies we use for stress management are helpful and sustainable. Self-harm, binge eating, excessive drinking, smoking, and recreational drug use are all maladaptive coping mechanisms. Maladaptive stress responses give us temporary relief but also do us harm. Ultimately, these tools leave the root issue unresolved, free to continually stress us.[1] We don't need to judge ourselves if we use these tools to cope with stress, but we do need to ask ourselves if these tools are serving us. Do these tools feel sustainable? Cultural messaging has taught many of us to prioritize the needs of everything and everyone else before our bodies or ourselves. Because of our programming, accepted behaviors, like dosing our frustration and sadness with rich food until we are paralyzed by the itis, might feel more approachable than taking a full mental health day. Give yourself permission to explore what needs are hiding behind destructive coping habits.

On the other hand, self-care is an excellent way to manage our stress. Self-care encompasses any behavior we engage in that is good for our body and soul. Nurturing our body and spirit requires us to show ourselves compassion and give ourselves care when we need it. Self-care requires spending time and effort to rejuvenate ourselves as whole beings. Self-care doesn't have to take the form of spa days, massages, and pedicures. Any practice that helps us manage our stress and promote our well-being is valid. This could include putting aside time for things that bring us joy, like grooming ourselves, spending time in silence, enjoying time in nature, and prioritizing rest.

The body gives us a wealth of information about how to nurture ourselves. The body cues us to address not only physical needs but our emotional ones as well. Learning to be present and understand the meaning behind the feelings we experience in our bodies gives us insight into where we need to pay more attention. Consciously tuning in to the body isn't just about experiencing pleasure; it's also about developing the ability to feel all of the sensations in the body, both pleasant and unpleasant. Developing a tolerance for simply sitting with uncomfortable feelings instead of immediately practicing avoidance is very helpful. Learning to face our feelings and trust our bodies and ourselves protects us from developing dependences on maladaptive tools that help us avoid uncomfortable feelings.

Eating when you are hungry and stopping when you are comfortably satisfied is self-care as much as taking a day off from the gym when you are physically exhausted.

Loving your body twenty-four hours a day every day is neither a necessary nor a realistic goal. Body autonomy is the goal. You should be the one calling the shots about your body. You decide when to share your body. You choose how to dress your body. No one has any business policing your body. Body policing covers everything from unsolicited comments about your weight to speculations about your gender-affirming surgery. Your body is your business. You don't need permission to be yourself. No opinion is more important than the one you have of yourself. Learning to nurture yourself is healthful in neutral spaces but crucial in hostile environments. The concept of self-care is simple but can present some challenges for people who have been socialized to ignore their needs.

JOURNALING BREAK

Let's assess where you are with self-care.

Reflect on the following statements. Journal your responses and any thoughts or feelings that come up for you.

I take time every day to do something I enjoy.

_____

_____

_____

I wear gender-affirming clothes that make me feel good about myself.

_____

_____

_____

I eat what I want when I want, in the quantities I want.

_____

_____

_____

_____

I don't allow myself to be coerced into eating beyond the point of fullness or into skipping seconds when I am hungry.

_____

_____

_____

_____

I create an eating environment that makes me feel relaxed and safe.

_____

_____

_____

I don't force myself to eat foods I don't enjoy because of perceived health benefits.

_____

_____

_____

I decline invitations when I feel overextended.

_____

_____

_____

It is easy for me to perceive the difference between thirst and hunger.

_____

_____

_____

I can easily identify things about myself that are lovable.

_____

_____

_____

These statements encompass more than just food, because learning to practice self-care is holistic and must extend beyond food. Eating is simply our entry point to learning to habitually take care of our needs.

PROTECTING YOUR PEACE

Mindfulness is an effective stress management tool for most people and has been shown to be helpful in mitigating minority stress as well.[2] Bullying and microaggressions related to gender expression, sexual orientation, or skin color can cause rumination and depressive symptoms. Staying grounded in the present helps limit the amount of time a traumatic incident involving bigotry can wear on us. It behooves us to adopt coping strategies that address both our external environment and our internal world. Individual-based strategies, like mindfulness, can be leveraged no matter what we have access to when it comes to support in our external environment.

Mindful eating, in particular, is a powerful tool because it's primed to be habit-forming, building on a natural part of our daily life. Instead of adding to all of the obligations we already have, mindful eating is simply making a modification to something we are already going to do several times a day. See mealtime as an opportunity to affirm your sense of self. Identify what you value and look for ways to structure mealtime in a way that is meaningful to you.

So often, when we are encouraged to pursue healthy habits, we are advised to push through resistance. We're told that even if developing a healthy habit is arduous or time-consuming, we should do it in anticipation of future benefits. But under the stress of daily life, healthy habits that promise to help us down the road tend to crumble. The wonderful thing about mindful eating is that many of the benefits are immediate. The practice guides you to eat in a way that is most pleasurable to you. Your digestion can immediately improve when you eat in a mindful way. The amount of satisfaction you get out of every mealtime increases in real time. What a delicious exercise! You get the benefits now *and* later.

Many of us have been socialized to believe that we cannot meet our needs on our own. However, the truth is you already know what you need to do to make your mealtimes nourishing rather than diminishing. The process of using nutrition as a self-care tool starts before mealtime. When you are shopping, consider which foods you enjoy the most. Thinking of all of your senses, which food will delight you? What sounds do you love hearing in the kitchen? What smells make your mouth water? Identify the foods you enjoy the most. Prioritize these as you plan out your meals. As you meal-plan, think of the textures, sounds, and aromas you most want to experience. Mealtimes themselves should be edifying and nourishing. When you are eating, try to identify any thoughts you have that contradict the fact that you are able to nourish yourself properly using your intuitive wisdom. Avoid looking for outside information to determine whether or not an item is "healthy" and good to consume freely. Focus instead on how you feel when you eat.

Bring mindfulness to the entire process of eating. Ideally, it is best to eat in a calm, quiet setting where you can digest your food with ease at your desired pace. But that isn't always possible during the workday or in a crowded, noisy household. Eating mindfully, however, isn't just for people who are able to eat in a serene environment. Once you set the intention to be aware of what you are eating and how your body is enjoying it, you will be able to start practicing eating in a mindful way.

Set the goal of staying in the moment throughout mealtime. Let the tastes, textures, and smells of your food anchor you to the present. It might be challenging to approach eating in a mindful way if you are accustomed to eating very quickly. Giving yourself the time to be observant and engage all of your senses in the eating process takes patience. When you first start this practice, try journaling during your meal to slow yourself down and encourage nonjudgmental awareness. There is generally a thirty-minute delay between when you start eating and when you begin to feel satisfied.[3] If you eat really rapidly, it's difficult to notice when you are approaching the point of satisfaction, so focusing your attention on slowing down will make it easier for you to feel when your physical hunger has been satisfied.

JOURNALING BREAK

Answering the following questions at your next meal will help you pace yourself.

Did I start to salivate at the thought of having this food?

_____

_____

_____

Would I say this food is one of my favorites?

_____

_____

_____

Why did I choose what I am eating for this meal?

_____

_____

_____

_____

How does the food feel in my mouth?

_____

_____

_____

Do I like this texture?

_____

_____

_____

Is there something I could change to make this more pleasurable (e.g., cook with less moisture, make it more crisp, cook it longer at a lower temperature for a softer texture)?

_____

_____

_____

Where did I sense the flavors in my mouth when the food first touched my tongue?

_____

_____

_____

How would I describe the flavor of the food to someone who has never tried this dish?

_____

_____

_____

Did the meal hit the spot as I thought it would?

_____

_____

_____

Is there something missing I could add right now to make this even better (e.g., hot sauce, fish sauce, vinegar, garlic powder)?

_____

_____

_____

Would it be possible to add that the next time I eat this?

_____

_____

_____

Think of your favorite food memory. Who was cooking? How did you feel when you ate the meal? Have you been able to recreate this experience since? Almost everyone has a food memory that has stuck with them for a lifetime. The memories of that meal stay with us because, at the time of the meal, we were fully present. Experiencing our food and allowing it to ground us in the present moment adds pleasure to the eating experience. It also allows us to exercise our mindfulness muscles. Frequently, our greatest food memories are linked to other people. When we eat in a communal environment, we are more likely to be present than if we are alone with our minds wandering, with our cell phone in hand. All of our power and agency is in the present tense. We cannot change the past, and we cannot control what happens in the future. The present is all we have. Allowing mealtimes to ground us serves us throughout the day. Being present helps us reduce our experience of stress and anxiety as we focus on what is directly in front of us instead of being caught in cycles of worry and regret. We can use food to build our ability to experience joy and stay present.

SENSING YOUR SATISFACTION

After you finish eating, continue your line of inquiry. How does your stomach feel? How would you describe your level of fullness on a scale from one to ten, one being hungry or ravenous and ten being stuffed to the gills? If you could have a do-over, would you have stopped eating earlier? Were you aware you were starting to get full prior to stopping? What stops you or discourages you from putting your fork down when you are beginning to feel full but you still have a few bites left? What beliefs do you have about food waste? If you sense an unhelpful belief about food waste, how can you reframe this belief to be a statement that still resonates with you as true but doesn't push you to eat beyond the point of fullness?

Introspection and intuition are the keys to this process. There is no need to strive for perfection. Do not pressure yourself to eat mindfully and consciously every single time you eat. This is a practice that we're going to lean into and use the majority of the times we eat. Any time we set an intention and continually refocus our attention, we will inevitably make progress. We don't have to force this process along. We don't have to make this hard. This entire process can be joyful. When we use food as a self-care tool, we are eating with the goal of nourishing ourselves. Eating in this way allows us to fully enjoy our food as we stay in the present moment and carefully observe our experience without judgment.

You'll be able to eat without guilt as you confirm throughout the meal that you are eating in response to a need. Instead of monitoring yourself for missteps, you are searching for greater enjoyment and a deeper experience of food. For example, instead of beating yourself up for eating beyond the point of fullness, just mark the experience. Acknowledge, accept, and forgive that you ate beyond the point of fullness and it made you feel uncomfortably stuffed. Clearly state your preferred feeling. Try to visualize and recall the physical sensations associated with that preferred stopping point. Over time, you will notice old habits that don't feel good for you falling away.

In the beginning, I recommend trying to eat with awareness at least once a day. Many people also engage in prayer or some acknowledgment of their ancestors or their higher self at mealtime. If this feels right to you, do it. If this resonates with you, connect or ground yourself, express gratitude, and set the intention to have the meal fuel and support you before your first bite. Ask for support in using this meal to show gratitude for your physical body and gratitude for the gift of intuition. Once you express that gratitude, it will help you stay connected to your goal of using this meal to both take care of your physical form and your emotional well-being.

Give yourself time to tune into how your body is responding to the food you are eating. This is an essential part of the process. Your body is the boss. Listen to it.

TRUSTING YOUR BODY

*Think with
the whole body.*

—Taisen Deshimaru

Your existence is a testament to the body wisdom of your
ancestors. You exist because your ancestors' bodies had the
wisdom to keep them alive in hostile and friendly environments alike.

Not only is your body more qualified than your conscious
mind to take care of your physiological needs, your body is
infinitely more informed about what you need to thrive than the
companies trying to sell you solutions to your supposed weight
problems. Your body has a vested interest in its own preservation. You don't need external help to know when and how deeply
to inhale. You don't need external guidance to figure out when to

urinate. Your body is equally capable of regulating energy needs. When your body requires more energy, it sends you signals to eat. When your body has what it needs, it sends you signals to stop eating.

Accepting that your body is fully capable of taking care of you without outside help might be difficult after so many years of being told that the body cannot be trusted. To further complicate things, if you have been ignoring your body for a long time, hearing what signals your body is sending will be a skill you'll have to rebuild.

JOURNALING BREAK

Try this exercise to start working toward getting in tune with your body's signals.

Pick a day when you don't have a lot on your agenda, preferably a quiet weekend at home.

Journal your observations before and after every meal and snack (use the space provided here and in a separate journal, if needed).

Try to sense what changes and how you feel just before you decide to eat.

Does your stomach feel empty?

_____

_____

_____

Does it growl?

_____

_____

_____

Do you feel light-headed? Do you feel cranky? Do you feel tired? Do you feel weak?

_____

_____

_____

Were you hit with a sudden, urgent need to eat?

_____

_____

_____

Did you have a specific craving?

_____

_____

_____

If you start to feel headachy, light-headed, or agitated before you eat, this means you missed the first signs of hunger. Hunger ebbs and flows. If you don't eat when you are first sent a hunger signal (often felt in the stomach), the hunger will temporarily subside. You are sent waves of hunger, and if you continue to ignore them, that is when you start feeling light-headed and cranky. Of course, there are exceptions to this rule. If you have a medical condition that affects your diet, you might have uniquely intense cues. I'm talking about the general population that doesn't have a diagnosed problem with regulating blood sugar. Remember that if you live with a food-related diagnosis, you should consult your physician or dietitian before making any changes to your diet.

When you are hit with emotional hunger, it's intense and sudden. When you are emotionally hungry, you are more likely to have a specific craving. Physical hunger can be satisfied with a variety of different tastes and textures; when you are driven to eat in response to emotional hunger, feelings of satiety escape you. You are pushed to eat beyond physical fullness.

Now, record how you feel after eating.

Do you feel satisfied?

_____

_____

_____

Are you uncomfortably full?

_____

_____

_____

Do you feel energized?

_____

_____

_____

Do you feel tense or relaxed?

_____

_____

_____

Do you feel regretful or guilty?

_____

_____

_____

On your journaling day, try to focus on really feeling your hunger signals. When you sit down to eat, eat slowly enough to sense the moment of satisfaction. You can use pleasure as your guide. As you approach satisfaction, the taste of your food becomes less intense. If you have ever eaten three pieces of cake in one sitting, you know that at some point during the third piece, you couldn't really taste the cake as you did on bite one.

Remember that it is also normal to eat for reasons aside from physical hunger. Our goal isn't to judge our motivation for eating. This journaling day is about observation. You absolutely don't have to do this every time you eat. This is just an exercise to explore your hunger and satiety cues.

HUNGER AS A KEY TO PLEASURE

If you note that you were not hungry prior to eating, observe how this affects your eating experience. Note the difference eating before experiencing physical hunger makes to satisfaction. Notice how food tastes and smells when you eat in the absence of physical hunger. Do you find satiety elusive? Do you feel more likely to continue eating beyond the point of fullness? Which sensations do you prefer? In an ideal situation, how would you prefer to handle the desire to eat in the absence of physical hunger in the future? In hindsight, were you able to identify what emotional state you were pursuing when you looked to food in the absence of physical hunger? Is there a way you could have filled your emotional needs in a more long-lasting, satisfactory way?

JOURNALING BREAK

If you still feel compelled to eat once you notice you are no longer hungry, try answering some of the following questions and see if any helpful insights come up for you.

What story am I telling myself right now about food waste?

_____

_____

_____

_____

What story am I telling myself about scarcity?

_____

_____

_____

_____

What feeling am I pursuing by continuing to eat beyond the point of fullness?

_____

_____

_____

_____

What stories do I tell myself about my value?

_____

_____

_____

_____

_____

Am I allowed to take a break?

_____

_____

_____

_____

_____

Do I have to be busy at all times?

_____

_____

_____

_____

_____

Am I eating in response to exhaustion and the need for downtime that I won't allow myself?

_____

_____

_____

_____

Will I consider it loving to continue eating once I feel overly full thirty minutes from now?

_____

_____

_____

_____

It's not possible or necessary to respond "correctly" to each and every one of our bodies' cues. Perfection is not the goal. Your body is an expert at achieving balance. If you let your body lead you, you will end up in a balanced place.

For now, let's just agree that you'll stop talking back to your body when it tells you what you need. Don't answer with "You just ate" when it says it's hungry or "I don't have time to listen to you right now" when it screams it is tired. If you keep ignoring the messages your body sends you, they will get harder to hear.

If you have been dieting for years, fear may come up when you think about trusting your body. You naturally wonder what will happen if you stop eating in a restrictive way and are left to your own devices. You may worry that you're not capable of self-regulating, that you will lose control of yourself when you give yourself permission to eat freely. The truth is it is very rare for the body's intuitive signals to become defective and untrustworthy. What you have to reconcile is what your body wants and needs and what your brain wants as a result of living in the misogynistic, white supremacist, homophobic, and transphobic soup, which may not always match up.

HEALING HUNGER TRAUMA

Growing up, my family was not food-insecure, but we were in a lower-income household, and we rarely, if ever, had unlimited access to seconds. Our family tradition was that whoever finished first was the one who got to have seconds. Because of that pattern, "grab it and growl" became the words to live by. Even though we were never in any danger of going hungry, plowing through our meals to get a second serving of our favorite foods became a ritual. As an adult, I continued to rush through meals and eat beyond the point of fullness because of that deeply ingrained pattern. I kept eating things before I wanted them, thinking on some level that they might not be available later. With work, I replaced that mantra with "I have enough. I always have enough." I know this is not unique to me. Many of us have suffered some form of food insecurity in our youth, which absolutely affects how we relate to eating and trusting our bodies as adults.

As you work toward accepting yourself, you will find it easier to accept that body diversity is just as natural and beautiful as all the types of diversity we observe in the human family. It is easy to be fooled into believing that you are not worthy when you are inundated by messaging that undermines you. Once you learn to question your assumptions, once you know to question your desire to be a specific size, you'll find it easier to distinguish between your body signals based on a physiological need and desire and your desires based on social programming.

Reframing eating as a tool for self-care that you do for the sake of feeling good as opposed to a way to control your body is powerful. When you use body-led eating instead of external cues, you free yourself to enjoy your food without guilt and focus on nourishing and pampering yourself by giving your body just the right amount of what it needs.

In pampering ourselves and showing ourselves love, we need to be on the lookout for neglected needs that present as emotional hunger. Eating when we aren't hungry is so common because eating in the absence of hunger has a numbing effect on the body. When you're totally overwhelmed and stressed out, bingeing is a way to stop yourself from feeling anything. Living and fighting with systems of oppression is exhausting. It only makes sense that marginalized folks need breaks and are often drawn to binge eating as a coping mechanism. Wanting to not feel anything in response to physical and mental beatdowns is a normal response to systemic oppression. When the pain is just too much, overeating leaves you feeling sedated. This is a useful short-term coping mechanism. But the problem is the effect doesn't last. When you eat in the absence of true hunger, no amount of food will satisfy you. This is why emotional hunger binges usually end with us uncomfortably full. It is natural to use food for more than just physical hunger; just be aware of its limits. If you have a pattern of eating in response to stress or eating to distract yourself, consider exploring what you are really hungry for.

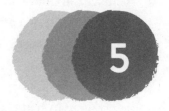

LIBERATING YOURSELF FROM BODY SHAME

It took many years of vomiting up all the filth I'd been taught about myself and half-believed before I was able to walk on the earth as though I had a right to be here.

—James Baldwin

Body shame: the persistent feeling that the body is flawed, inadequate, and in need of correction

The American dream boils down to the pursuit of wealth and privilege. Even though it isn't advertised as the predominant faith, history clearly betrays the truth; here, we worship the almighty dollar. Anytime something exists in a pervasive way in the dominant culture, in the open market, or on major media outlets, it's because it generates massive amounts of money.

People have a soul. People have a conscience. In contrast, within corporations, companies, and groups, where individual people don't have to take responsibility for the actions of the whole, there is no conscience. It isn't logical to believe that companies want to take care of you or prioritize human happiness over profits.

The diet industry is not here to help you. The diet industry is not here to battle some imaginary healthcare crisis. The diet industry is here to take advantage of you and consume your resources. The diet industry commodifies the body and uses it to generate profit.

Refusing to allow your body to be commodified or used requires that you opt out of diet culture and reject the body shame it continually propagates. Reclaiming your body as exclusively your own is empowering, not just for your spirit and for your sense of self but for your wallet as well. These organizations are not worthy of your dollars. Upholding colonized concepts of beauty is not valuable on any level. Focusing on liberation is a far better use of your time and resources. Decolonization is a far better use of our time and resources. Decolonization is the work we do to untangle ourselves from all manifestations of white supremacy and heteronormativity. If you see yourself through the eyes of the colonizer, you base your value on your ability to live up to heteronormative and Eurocentric standards.

Clients frequently reflect back to me that their feelings of conflict around their bodies and gender presentations started very early in life. Let me share with you this account from one client in their own words:

"I first started really being body conscious and aware of my weight when I was really young and impressionable," says Jamal, a transmasculine person raised in the 1990s. "All those things like beauty standards and the media and everything played into the way I related to myself. It always felt bad, whether it was catalogs or movies, that there was never someone who looked like me. I could never relate to anyone I saw.

"I remember, when I was about six, the first moment my mom had to explain to me that I was a girl and that I couldn't do certain things boys could. As a kid, to me, my body was just like the boys'; you know, at the time, our bodies were relatively similar. I had all guy friends in my neighborhood, and they would all run around shirtless, and they would be playing on their bikes, having their trucks, their G.I. Joes and stuff, and I would be out there right with them. And I took off my shirt. To me, we looked the same, and it didn't even cross my mind that I was different, that I was a different gender than them.

"My mom pulled me aside and was like, 'No, no, you gotta put your clothes on; you're a girl, and that's not ladylike,' and I'm over here with skinned knees, wearing baggy pants and not understanding the rules.

"I was nine when I told my mom I should have been born a boy. She said, 'Oh, we'll pray about it. You know God doesn't make mistakes. You are perfect just the way you are.' It just didn't feel right. She was like, 'You're just a tomboy.' And yeah, there's space for that, but for me, it was always more than that. Tomboys are aware that they are female, and they're fine with that. Being a masculine woman is different from being a transman. At that point, I knew something wasn't right. I just didn't know what the words were to explain it."

Most of us are not raised to believe that we are exclusively entitled to our bodies, that we can trust our gut and follow our heart. I've been told by countless individuals that they recognized their gender nonconformity in early childhood and were advised by adults and caretakers to ignore their inner wisdom and perform their assigned gender as dictated by the norms of their community of origin. This experience adds to the layers of socializing that encourages disconnect from the body.

RECLAIMING EMBODIMENT

In a different way, I also had suspicions that my body might be wrong before I started kindergarten. When my mom took me to orientation and parent after parent walked past me to fawn over the loosely coiled hair of fair-skinned students, those suspicions started to crystallize. At the age of five, I learned that nothing is more interesting than how a girl looks; being pretty (in a Eurocentric way, of course) was key to accessing popularity and value. Being dark-skinned and having tightly coiled hair made you invisible, too uninteresting, unglamorous, and unimportant to be acknowledged.

Despite internalizing negative messaging about my worth, I maintained high grades throughout school, graduating sixth in my class with a 3.8 grade point average. But I continued to be invisible. No teacher or counselor ever asked where I'd be attending school after graduation or if I needed any help or guidance with deciding what my next academic step might be.

When I decided to take courses at the community college my senior year of high school as a dual-enrolled student, I was stopped at least a few times a week as I came to campus to attend my high school classes at the end of the day. Now, I am not from a big city. I'm from a town where, even when I visit now, people

I've never met before greet and recognize me because I look like my mother and grandmother. I'd known most of the kids I graduated with since elementary school. The reason these teachers couldn't recognize me even though I'd seen them every day since freshman year was that their unresolved negative bias against dark skin and femme people made me all but invisible to them. Every time I was stopped, the assumption was that I was an underperforming student up to no good. No one ever assumed I was dual-enrolled. At first, I thought my invisibility was my fault, that maybe it was related to something I was doing. Maybe my low school spirit and nineties *Daria*-esque disposition weren't compelling. But as I saw how much attention C-average students with lighter complexions received, plus accolades and support from counselors and teachers, I got the message.

It took years of therapy and processing to identify and heal the damage that going to a school steeped in white supremacy and misogyny did to my spirit. The homophobia and white supremacy from my religious upbringing didn't do me any favors either. I share a little bit of my story with you to tell you that it is exceedingly common for people to spend a good portion of their adulthood processing and healing from their childhood. It isn't fair that any child is exposed to hurtful and unloving messaging, but it happens every day. The good news is we aren't kids anymore. We have agency. We have a say in what we are exposed to now. We can give ourselves the protection and consideration we always deserved but weren't given as children.

Shielding yourself from toxicity is self-care. Meanwhile, perfectionism and binary thinking are excellent fodder for shame. Stay on the lookout for these earmarks of white supremacy culture. Note when a reductionist view of wellness, gender expression, and your value as a human being are generating a sense of shame and malaise within you. Your body is meant to serve you and you only. It's helpful to spend some time getting clear on what you would like your relationship to your body to be like.

JOURNALING BREAK

Take some time to reflect on the following questions and journal your observations. Some people find it helpful to write these responses in the form of a letter addressed to their body.

What about my body do I appreciate right now? _____

_____

_____

_____

_____

In what ways does my body feel like home? _____

_____

_____

_____

_____

I feel disconnected from my body because _____

_____

_____

_____

_____

I hate my body because it has _____

_____

_____

_____

_____

I don't recognize my body because _____

_____

_____

_____

_____

I was comfortable in my body until _____

_____

_____

_____

_____

I was never fully aware of my body until _____

_____

_____

_____

_____

I would feel at home in my body if _____

_____

_____

_____

_____

_____

My body gives me access to _____

_____

_____

_____

_____

My body blocks me from accessing _____

_____

_____

_____

_____

I am angry at my body because _____

_____

_____

_____

_____

I feel betrayed by my body because _____

_____

_____

_____

_____

Once you start to clarify what your current perception of your body is, you will be able to see where you can start to improve your relationship with it. If you find that you resent your body because it locks you into living a false persona that doesn't match your gender identity, that is valid. It will be important for you to explore practices you can adopt now to help you feel more comfortable with the body you have at this moment. Freedom to present your authentic self is a key factor in wellness. Do not allow anyone to dissuade you from your truth. To the extent that is safe for you, please pursue authenticity ferociously. Being yourself is a gift to the world. Only you can determine what that will look like. Feel free to experiment and remember that you are allowed to change your mind as you go along. Don't worry about learning to express yourself authentically twenty-four seven. All you need to do is give yourself permission to be the decision maker for what is right for you and your body and see where that leads you.

Gender-affirming surgery is not the only tool at your disposal to align your gender expression with your truth. Finding an affirming physician who can advise you on safe ways to bind and inform you of all your options for accurate gender expression is incredibly helpful. Because reliable health care has been such a challenge for trans folks, people from within the gender nonconforming (GNC) community are developing resources to address this problem (see page 147).

GROUND YOURSELF

Breaking the chains of body shame will be both a solo and a communal activity. Developing a practice that helps you feel grounded in your body can be helpful in recovering the sense that it belongs to you and is not beholden to any external expectations. Embodiment exercises, moving meditations, and joyful movement can help with this. Embodiment exercises are a series of movements done to help you center your attention on sensations in the body. These can be very simple and can be done by yourself or with loved ones. Try the exercises below and see if any of these feel like they are for you.

Head-Carrying

Our posture frequently communicates a lot about our emotional state. Since standing erect and practicing a healthy posture while balancing weighted objects on your head requires attention, it's an excellent embodiment exercise.

Select an object or two that won't hurt you or be damaged if/ when it falls off your head. I generally recommend starting with a couple of books.

Stand with your feet shoulder-width apart if you are able. This exercise can also be done in a seated position if that is best for your body.

Press your feet into the floor. Focus on your big toe, feel it securely placed on the floor. Shift your focus to your smallest toe, then your heel. Once you feel stable at your base, start to relax your neck and shoulder muscles. Roll your shoulders back and keep your spine in a comfortable erect position. Place the weighted objects you have chosen on your head. Allow the tension in your upper body to unwind while maintaining your posture.

Feel your chest expanding as you settle into this position. Breathe as deeply as you can without losing your weighted objects, observing where you feel tension and where you feel comfortable with every breath.

Solo-Caress

In a position that is comfortable for you, vigorously rub the palms of your hands together. Once you feel the warmth they've generated, gently pull your hands apart and push them back together without allowing them to touch. Pay close attention to the sensations you observe in your hands as you do this. Place your hands on your neck, then on your face. Stroke any parts of your body that feel neutral to you (e.g., wrists, collarbone) and really notice them. Caress, appreciate, and observe how these parts of your body feel in the moment. If you are comfortable, extend this to your arms and torso. Stroke your body as you would if you were applying shea butter or a body cream.

Joyful Movement

Joyful movement is exercise reframed. Exercise is helpful in that it helps you stay grounded in your body. Even if you have a complicated relationship with your body, moving it in ways that feel playful and fun can be enriching. If you enjoy traditional forms of exercise, that is fine. Joyful movement for you might be trail running, but for most people, joyful movement will look more like play.

What ways do you move your body just for fun? Informal dance is an extremely popular choice for joyful movement. You don't have to set up an elaborate opportunity to dance, and you don't have to make this difficult or complicated. You might find that dancing in your bedroom or while you're doing dishes brings you joy. If you love dancing and community then consider partner dancing or dancing in a group setting. If you feel more comfortable dancing in your own bedroom with the door locked, then do that. It's very important that whatever form of movement you choose, it needs to be your idea, based on what you had a strong feeling you would enjoy.

I have never felt like a strong or talented dancer, but I kept feeling tempted to check out the African dance classes offered in Atlanta. I'd heard there were live drums. I worried I wouldn't learn the steps quickly enough and I would feel like an ass for trying something new. Eventually, my desire to check out a class with live drums overcame my fear of embarrassment and I went to my first class. It was breathtaking. I didn't learn the steps quickly, and yes, the seven- and nine-year-olds showed me up, but it was so invigorating to be in a space centered on celebrating the African diaspora that none of that mattered. The dance classes I attend focus on the traditional significance of dance as a form of storytelling. Perfection is not required. Everyone experiences the movements in their own way. If you can't remember the last time you had fun moving your body, reference your childhood. If you suggest a game of hopscotch or double Dutch, you might be surprised how many of your friends would want to get in on that.

CLEAN OUT YOUR CLOSET

To liberate yourself from body shame, you also need to look for items in your home that reveal your longing for the body you used to have instead of thoroughly enjoying the body you have at this moment. Even after accepting that dieting doesn't work and definitely isn't a health-promoting behavior, you might find yourself clinging to clothes from when you were in a smaller body. Having those clothes will keep tempting you to strive for an externally determined weight instead of working on getting comfortable with allowing your body to guide you to a comfortable weight of its own choosing. Clinging to the idea of being a specific size is not at all helpful as you learn to eat according to your body's cues.

Every time you come across something in your home or life that triggers you to think that you need to force your body to shrink, get rid of it. Your body might naturally vary in size as you start tuning in to your own hunger. That is perfectly fine. In fact, your body changing size over time is a very natural process, and this can go in either direction. The danger is in trying to force your body to change. Nothing will make you feel like your body is wrong faster than wearing clothes that dig into you. Sizing is arbitrary, inconsistent, and can't tell you anything about your body's quality or acceptability. Wear whatever size feels comfortable on your body and doesn't punishingly dig into you. Resist the temptation to buy clothes that almost fit.

What message are you sending to yourself when you wear clothes that make you feel anything less than comfortable? As a child, I remember dreading having to wear at least calf-length skirts, endless amounts of little frilly socks, and more pink than you could shake a stick at. There's nothing wrong with any of those things. They just weren't me.

As I moved closer to accepting that it is not only OK to be yourself, but it's a vital part of living your best life, cultivating contentment not just for you but for everyone around you, the more I gave myself permission to wear what I felt at home in.

The day I got rid of all of my dresses and skirts, I felt like a weight was lifted off my shoulders. I felt good in a way that

I could not have imagined before doing it. Just knowing that I don't ever have to wear a dress again makes me feel more at ease. It's hard to explain how significant it is to keep being asked to wear things that just don't feel like you.

"I always felt really uncomfortable in feminine clothes, almost like it was physically restrictive in some way," Jamal agrees. "Puberty was just about the death of me. All of a sudden I'm growing, bleeding, developing upstairs, and feeling like this is not OK, having to go bra shopping and being stuck in the girls' section, picking out stuff.

"First of all, I'm not shaped like most women. I'm tall, and I've always been a little bit bigger and, you know, plus-size sections weren't exactly a thing in the juniors' section. When my mom said, 'I guess you're too tall for the junior sizes, so we're going to go to women's,' I was just cringing on the inside. Finally, I somehow talked her into buying me men's clothes because they fit, and I was like, *Oh, I feel more confident in this because it fits my body and I'm shaped more like this, and it just feels better not having to wear something that's super feminine or even a tiny bit feminine.*"

Focus on editing your wardrobe to include only clothes that make you feel your best, clothes that fit comfortably and present you to the world in the way you would like to be seen. Prioritize finding gender-affirming clothing. However, if it is dangerous for you to present in a way that is comfortable for you, that's an understandable reason to make concessions. If that is a concern for you because of your gender presentation and where you live, consider safe ways you can feel more comfortable in your clothing and start looking for safe spaces and people to put around you as a buffer. You are the one who will ultimately have to decide how much you are willing to sacrifice being yourself. When you reach the point of being ready to be yourself no matter the cost, you will know it.

I love Marie Kondo's outlook on keeping only clothing that sparks joy.[1] She suggests that you hold each piece of clothing you own and sense if it sparks joy in you. If you find pieces in your wardrobe that don't light you up, let them go. This practice of checking in with how your body physically accepts or rejects clothing is so helpful for deciding what gender-affirming pieces to keep in your wardrobe. Take the clothes that no longer serve you and sell them online or pass them on to a friend. Consider throwing a clothing-swap party with your friend circle if buying new clothes isn't practical for you right now. You don't need to have an extensive wardrobe for it to give you joy. A capsule wardrobe with a few essential central pieces that you can build and combine with accessories is a smart, budget-friendly way to go. As you build a capsule wardrobe, you can purchase a minimum amount of items that really focus on versatility and things that suit you. You might find your next beloved piece at a secondhand shop or online consignment store. I look for central wardrobe pieces on sites that focus on gender-neutral clothes since that feels best to me. I make sure to buy these only in my favorite colors since a foundation wardrobe is all about versatility; you want to make sure your central pieces can be combined with most things you own. You can create virtual lookbooks for yourself using a site like Pinterest to pin things that fit your aesthetic. This will help you connect with other people who have a similar sense of style for more inspiration and lead you to brands that appeal to you.

SIDESTEP THE SHAME SPIRAL

Internalized racism, misogyny, and homophobia can feel embarrassing or shameful to acknowledge, but you can't remove something you can't see. We have to face and accept what is in order to remove it from ourselves and start healing. Shame is not a productive emotion, but it is natural, so please don't start feeling ashamed of your shame. We live in a racist, homophobic, and heteronormative world. These biases are atmospheric. It's only natural that we've all been tainted by these beliefs. The good news is once you become aware of your internalized biases, you can free yourself from them. Untangling our complicated relationship to our bodies and food is a very tangible way to start working on our sense of self-worth and self-efficacy.

Cisgender, het white folks have the benefit of being immersed in messages and images that promote a positive sense of self, if not at least a neutral one. Even though we might not have this unearned privilege, with awareness and planning, we can shield ourselves from media that undermines us and press ahead on our journey to total liberation.

Ultimately, body liberation is about freeing yourself from the commodification of your body, rejecting the use of your body as a tool of capitalism, and claiming your freedom. It's about abandoning colonized ideas of acceptability and reclaiming the freedom to live your life on your terms and use your body as a vehicle for your pleasure and exploration of the world.

We live in an environment that encourages us to obsess over individual parts of the body. We are taught to pick ourselves apart and look for ways to "fix" our bodies one piece at a time. The beauty standards we are presented with by mainstream media elevate thin, white, cis, feminine beauty as the pinnacle. When we see one white cis-female celebrity lauded for her beautiful legs and another for her toned arms, we are being trained to idealize individual parts of the body. The beauty standard is elusive by design. It is meant to generate a sense of deficit and inadequacy in us so we will be motivated to buy products that promise to fix us. When we start to look at every little piece of ourselves as something to be scrutinized instead of living in the truth that we are whole beings, we can't help but fall down into a pit of self-criticism toward low self-image.

Respect and appreciate the body as a whole. Do not participate in your own exploitation. Avoid toxic messaging that reduces the body to parts. Untangling yourself from internalized negative messaging is a process. It took years for society to teach you to reject yourself. It's unrealistic to think that it won't take an ongoing effort to free yourself. The good news is you can shift the way you see yourself.

Healing your internalized biases will help you return to what you knew as an infant: you are enough. You are worthy of love and don't need to lift a finger to prove your value. The truth is the tools you need to live a free life are within you. We are trained to forget our intrinsic worth. If you have ever witnessed the utter confidence with which an infant can fill a diaper in a crowded room with no hint of shame, you know what I mean. An infant has to be taught shame. An infant is taught that taking a dump in a crowded room is a social faux pas.

We are born naturally convinced of our own goodness. Some of us were slowly brainwashed into believing we were less than, some of us had that beaten into us, and some of us stopped believing in our worth after years of sexual abuse. No matter what you have survived, you can find your way back to that place of self-love. Learning to feel safe enough in your body and relax into feeling its cues might require therapy-assisted work if, to protect you, your body lowered its sensitivity. As a survival strategy, the wise human body often goes numb (sometimes for long periods) in response to trauma.[2] If this resonates with you, thank your body for doing what it took to guarantee your survival. You are in this together, and you always have been. Together, you will work on regaining sensitivity, learning to hear and respect your body's cues as you once did.

LOOKING WITHIN

Tarot and oracle cards are accessible divination tools that can be used to connect you to your true desires and subconscious thoughts. Using tarot as a daily journaling prompt is an extremely powerful way to connect with and reflect on messages your higher self is sending you. Once you have worked through the exercises in this book, I highly recommend establishing a daily practice that will support your ongoing growth. Complete a reading for yourself and see if this daily practice is the one for you.

The process is simple. Shuffle the deck a few times. Ask what you need to know right now to stay in alignment and manifest greater freedom in your life. Spread the cards and select a single card. Look at the card itself and observe what initial feelings or thoughts come up for you. What stands out to you? Jot down your initial impressions. After you reflect on what message the card may hold for you, use the guidebook that came with your deck for a general interpretation of the card. Does that meaning connect to your initial feelings? Journal the connections between your life right now and the card. Answer any questions that came up in the guidebook or while you were reflecting on the card. Use your intuition. Don't edit yourself; go with your initial impressions. This journaling practice partners very well with a grounding practice.

LOVING KINDNESS MEDITATION

Sitting in stillness or meditating is a practical way to ground yourself and connect to sensing shifts in the body in real time. Instead of trying to force or shame yourself into self-compassion, you can try a simple meditation without expectations. If you stick with the practice, you may find yourself shifting over time.

There is no wrong way to meditate. It is all about personal preference. There are several resources on body awareness meditations, mantra meditations, and movement meditations that you might find useful for reconnecting to the body and increasing your self-compassion. Don't worry if the first practices you try don't resonate with you. There are plenty to choose from. Here is a simple meditation to get you started.

Sit comfortably. Don't force your body into a position. Honor your body's comfort. Try to open your chest by moving your shoulder blades toward each other comfortably. Rest both hands over your heart. Read each line below silently. Close your eyes. Breathe the sentence in. Visualize breathing the words into the center of your chest, into your heart. Repeat the line silently, take a deep breath, and exhale fully before moving to the next line. Without judgment, try to notice any areas in the body that are numb.

May I be safe and protected from inner and outer harm.

May I be free of mental pain and suffering.

May I be happy.

May I be free of physical pain and suffering.

May I be able to live in this world happily, peacefully, joyfully, and with ease.

May I care for myself.

May all of the world's queer children be safe, happy, and free from suffering.

May all trans folks be safe.

May all trans folks be happy.

May all Black, Indigenous, and people of color be safe, happy, healthy, and free from suffering.

May all beings be happy.

6

PRIORITIZING PLEASURE

To burn with desire and keep quiet about it is the greatest punishment we can bring on ourselves.
— Federico García Lorca, "Blood Wedding,"
in *Blood Wedding and Yerma*

When the world is withholding affection, we can't pass up opportunities to indulge and pamper ourselves. Focusing on pleasure is a joyful alternative to self-denial and martyrdom. Pleasure is often not prioritized by marginalized people in a conscious way. If you have received messaging that you are not deserving of pleasure or that your needs aren't worthy of being prioritized when you do pursue pleasure, you may be inclined to do it in a clandestine way, as though you are taking something that isn't rightfully yours.

Pleasure is a powerful communication tool your body uses to tell you you're doing the right thing. There are several examples of nature using a pleasurable response to encourage you to do something fundamental for the survival of the species. We don't have to worry about the human population dwindling to nothing because the "work" of procreating comes with pleasurable feedback. That is no accident. In the wild, things that are unsafe for human consumption often have an off-putting, bitter taste that prompts you to spit them out as soon as they touch your tongue. Pleasure is one of nature's favorite cues. Let's tap into this natural resource and allow ourselves to be guided by it when we nourish ourselves.

Pleasure can accurately inform what, when, and how much you should eat. Looking for your body to experience ease and pleasure is an excellent cue to search for. What a fun project, learning how to eat in the way that is most pleasurable to you.

JOURNALING BREAK

Here is an exercise to get you started. Buy a little stash of one of your favorite snacks. Over the course of the day or a couple of days, eat this snack (1) when you aren't physically hungry but the snack sounds good to you, (2) when you are sure you are physically hungry, and (3) at the end of a meal.

Each time, chew your snack slowly enough to savor it. Journal what you notice.

Is the taste intensely satisfying? _____

_____

_____

_____

Is the taste muted? _____

_____

_____

_____

Did it hit the spot? _____

_____

_____

_____

Notice how you experience your favorite snack differently depending on your hunger levels. After you have done all three tests, ask yourself when the snack was most delicious.

If you eat with the goal of truly indulging yourself each time, eating for reasons other than physical hunger starts to lose its appeal. The first few bites of cake are the most delightful. A bowl of soup is the most satisfying when you sit down to enjoy it after hunger has hit you. There is a reason why portions served in fine dining are so small. The objective is to give patrons an intensely pleasurable sensory experience with each course. This is best achieved with small portions, taste buds that aren't exhausted, and carefully designed flavor experiences that can be relished.

Eating when you aren't hungry gives you a muted, substandard experience of the food. As we discussed, eating when you aren't hungry can be a strong coping tool when you are looking for numbness to shelter yourself from extreme pain. If you find yourself eating and stuffing yourself when you aren't hungry, looking for a feeling of satisfaction that never comes, you aren't eating because you love food. You are eating to fill another need.

You are hungry for something else. There is nothing shameful about this habit. Your body is turning to a coping tool that it knows has protected you in the past. The problem with this tool is that it isn't meant for long-term use. It doesn't address your actual need. It is just a Band-Aid. Genuine kindness and self-care involve giving yourself the love and attention you truly need and feeding your spirit what it needs to be nourished and healed. You wouldn't offer a child a popsicle and nothing else if they came to you with a scraped knee. Give yourself the kindness you deserve. Feed your spirit what it actually needs.

Unfortunately, there is no magical tool for dealing with pain that doesn't involve confronting and experiencing your feelings. As miserable and difficult as it is to process a feeling, you have to experience it. Stuffing your feelings down with food doesn't get rid of them; it just suppresses them, leaving them in your body to fester. Finding a good therapist who respects and celebrates your marginalized identities is priceless in learning how to process pain and trauma. One of the greatest tools I gained from therapy was learning how to self-validate. Naming your emotion, giving yourself permission to feel your feelings without judgment, and affirming that your feelings are valid and acceptable stops you from compounding negative feelings with self-judgment. It is exceedingly common for marginalized folks (people of color in particular) to be subjected to years of conditioning that says it isn't safe or acceptable to be angry. Expressing pain is often seen as weak or unproductive. We have been trained to undermine or undervalue strong emotions when they arise. Your knee-jerk reaction to feeling hurt might be to tell yourself that it's stupid or pointless to feel that way. That is invalidating your feelings as a result of training. Accepting and validating your emotions is crucial to being able to work with and move through them. In addition to therapy, mindfulness and meditation practices that teach you how to sit with uncomfortable feelings can be powerful (see pages 74–79 and 99–102).

Beyond arising from with the stress of pain from past traumas or current emotional abuse from the world around us, emotional hunger can also come from neglecting the things in life that bring you joy. There is something very sad about moving through the world as an invisible person whose needs are rarely considered and even less frequently addressed. It can be challenging to find the words to explain this concept without stories or specific examples of what it feels like to go through life feeling hindered or dismissed, then coming into a rare experience where you feel genuinely welcome.

Let me give you a personal example. I am a spa person. Luxury is one of my core desires (more on this later). I feel like I'm living my best life when I do something that is 100 percent for me, and there is no reason to do it other than to give myself pleasure. As such, I enjoy getting massages and indulgent spa treatments. What I don't appreciate is paying for these experiences and then having to deal with microaggressions that do not support my desire to relax or feel indulged. The annoyances I've encountered most frequently are frigid treatment in the waiting room, having to wait as employees scramble to find acceptable products for tightly coiled hair, and having someone repeatedly pull my wild and lovely hair out of the way with a wimpy hair tie that's suited for either bone-straight hair or very loose curls, which continually pops off during the spa treatment. None of these experiences contribute to the luxe feeling I pay for, which other paying clients seem to be consistently getting. Each incident is a reminder that no one was expecting me and I am an unwelcome guest.

People of color and LGBTQIA+ folks are not often able to pick any place at random and feel confident that no one will be surprised to see them and people there will welcome them. Observing yet another manifestation of being pushed to the margins didn't devastate me. It simply gave me the clarity I needed to create an ultimate spa experience for myself as a person of color. When I lay down and started to get situated for my massage during my first visit to a Black-owned spa, the masseuse deftly swept up my hair between her fingers and did a quick braid that stayed in place for the duration of the treatment. I was not prepared for the wave of emotion that came over me. In an instant, I felt safe and at home. I was a welcomed guest. Knowing that my Blackness was neutral, welcomed, and expected in that space allowed me to relax into the best spa experience of my life. I hadn't realized until then that I never had been able to fully relax in other spaces, that other spaces hadn't felt safe, that I had been shortchanged and deprived of the luxe experience I had been seeking. Once I felt confident that I could focus on my own experience and enjoy the massage without bracing for the next microaggression, I felt the tension in my muscles melt away.

CORE DESIRES

Let's try to identify what some of *your* core desires are. What makes you feel satisfied and safe? What grounds you in the present moment and consistently gives you joy? Of course, there are a ton of variations when it comes to this sort of thing, so here is a list to get your wheels turning:

- Connecting with others
- Time alone
- Idle time (for daydreaming or puttering around the house)
- Quality time with family
- Personal freedom
- Luxury and indulgence
- A rich spiritual life
- Time in nature
- Intellectual growth
- Personal development
- Feeling understood by others
- A sense of order
- Adventure
- Having time to relish anticipation (e.g., reading menus days before you visit a restaurant, enjoying thinking about vacation more than being on vacation)
- Physical activity
- Intimacy
- Laughter
- Enjoying music
- Taking care of others
- Being recognized for your talents or accomplishments
- Structured time/having an itinerary
- Free time

Look at the list and sense what seems true to you. See how it feels in your body when you say:

"I need . . ."

"I don't feel right unless I have . . ."

"I will give myself . . ."

If you feel light, then you know you're on to something and this is something you need. This is one of your core desires, something you hunger for.

When you find a core craving or desire, don't deprive yourself of it. Make plans to feed it. If you are having trouble recognizing your core desires, check with a trusted friend. It will be easy for them to point out what they see you seeking out. Make sure you only do this activity with someone whose opinion you appreciate and respect, with someone you can safely disagree with. You need the freedom to throw out anything that doesn't resonate with you. This is about you and your needs. In a world that is rarely kind, you deserve pleasure. You deserve a delicious life.

JOURNALING BREAK

Try out these affirmations and journal any thoughts that come up. If these statements feel fake or uncomfortable and you can't connect to them, modify your affirmations to include "I'm learning to . . ."

I put a high value on indulgence and desire.

_____

_____

_____

_____

I honor my love of pampering myself and indulging in things on my terms at mealtimes.

_____

_____

_____

_____

I eat what I want.

_____

_____

_____

_____

I eat things that make me feel good physically and delight my senses.

_____

_____

_____

_____

I prefer monotasking and eating in a quiet spot.

_____

_____

_____

_____

I deliberately eat alone or choose my lunch partners carefully.

_____

_____

_____

_____

I control my environment and request changes when my desires aren't met.

_____

_____

_____

_____

Remember that you are entitled to feel pleasure throughout the day, and that includes mealtime. If your primary priority at this stage in your life is efficiency, maybe the idea of making dining pleasurable sounds like too much of a fuss to you. That is absolutely fine. There is no wrong way to do what works for you. The important thing is that you make sure you tailor things to you. Tune into what you desire and what you find valuable.

Let go of doing things out of a sense of obligation. Release suppressing your needs and cravings because someone told you to. Connecting to your physical and emotional hungers will open up a world of possibilities for you. Explore your body and take charge of your pleasure. There is no such thing as a "guilty pleasure." Pleasure is your divine right. There is nothing guilty about it.

LUXURIATING IN SELF-LOVE

If you can't love yourself, how in the hell are you gonna love somebody else?

—RuPaul

Focusing on yourself and your relationship to your body may seem like a luxury with so many pressing human rights issues to battle. But our sense of self-worth affects so many things that it cannot be ignored. If you are invested in the advancement and progress of your community, a strong sense of self-worth and a clear understanding of your intrinsic value are essential. Caring for ourselves puts us in a better position to advocate for others. Happiness and contentment are integral health-promoting aspects of life. The chronic low-grade stress that one experiences when being "othered" compromises emotional well-being and health. Being part of one marginalized group does not exempt you from additional abuse for other marginalized identities, making it difficult for some of us to find safe spaces or respites from psychological and physical abuse. Nurturing yourself protects your peace and energy. Self-love is a survival skill, not a luxury for the privileged.

It took you years to get to where you are right now, and it may take more time than you would like to start unraveling some of your inner conflicts. Be gentle with yourself. This isn't a race. There is no finish line. If anything, decolonization and the pursuit of body liberation is a daily practice. Hopefully, one day in the future, people who look and identify like us won't need to do serious emotional and psychological work to reverse the damage of years of abuse from their external environment, but from where I stand right now, that might be a while. So, realistically, as you continue to do your inner work, you'll continue to confront messaging that challenges your self-worth and undermines your pursuit of happiness. You can't control what other people think about you, but you can learn to set and reinforce boundaries. Save yourself the energy of deciding what to do each time you are confronted with a microaggression or blatant bigotry and hatred by setting personal policies. Of course, you can update these at any time, but already having a set of rules for how you deal with displays of white and hetero supremacy will save you massive amounts of emotional energy.

Look at this list of possible strategies and take note of any that resonate with you.

Rules of Engagement

1. Don't feed the trolls. When online, do not respond to or interact with internet bullies of any kind.

2. Get out of the free emotional labor business. Instead of guiding aspiring allies on their journey of personal improvement one-on-one, create opportunities for people to compensate you for your time and energy or direct them to the local library or a search engine.

3. Banish energy vampires. People who feign ignorance and request evidence or proof about the validity of our lived experiences are poison. When someone attempts to sap your energy by asking you to prove that systems of oppression are real or that a personal tale of discrimination isn't hyperbole, do not engage. No matter how innocent this person pretends to be, their gaslighting is a sly form of bullying. Don't allow them to continue undermining your experience. Confront them in a direct and straightforward way by saying, "I hear that you don't understand or relate to my experience; that doesn't mean it didn't happen," or "I don't need to prove my lived experience. I came to you for compassion. If you aren't able to offer me empathy, we don't need to have this conversation."

4. Call microaggressions out. Make it clear that you won't tolerate subtle forms of abuse. Simple responses like "I'm not comfortable with this," "Could you say more about what you mean by that?" "Please don't do that," or "This is not acceptable" are powerful and require no follow-up.

5. Leave toxic spaces. Feel free to leave virtual and physical spaces where you see problematic behavior with or without explanation.

TAKING BACK OUR POWER

Unchecked stress is a killer. Marginalized people need to be proficient at setting and maintaining boundaries and shielding ourselves from any stress we can potentially opt out of. Boundary-setting is a helpful tool, but we are rarely taught it. Our social conditioning is generally geared more toward tolerating abuse and stifling our voices to reduce our risk of facing violent retaliation. Using our voice, stepping into our power, and setting boundaries can be scary. Speaking up has meant death for countless ancestors. That collective trauma is real. But working through our fear and advocating for ourselves is empowering. Boundaries are the protective walls we use to create spaces where we feel safe enough to be our authentic selves. Because they allow us to set clear rules for what types of people and behaviors we allow in our lives, boundaries are the *foundation* of healthy relationships.

Standing up for ourselves and refusing to accept abuse from strangers and people in positions of power is challenging. Learning to set boundaries with family (particularly parents) is exceedingly difficult if you come from a background in which you are trained to never question or talk back to your elders. The first block you have to get past to step into using boundaries as a self-care tool is the misconception that you have to be harsh or mean to set and hold boundaries. Boundaries are simply how we communicate our limits and what kind of treatment we will or will not tolerate. It is entirely possible (but not mandatory) to say no with love in your heart. You don't need to bottle up your frustrations. You can respect the path of others while respecting yourself. When you clearly set limits, you aren't invalidating the will or beliefs of others; you are taking responsibility for your own well-being. Your feelings are just as important as the feelings of those around you. You don't need to tone-police yourself. You are free to express your limits in whatever way feels right for you. Speaking your truth early and often will help you feel in control of your environment. If you feel like your emotions are erupting when you confront a microaggression, it could be an indicator that you haven't been setting and reinforcing your boundaries often enough. Speaking up for yourself without delay stops frustration from mounting.

Initially, it might feel awkward or uncomfortable to stand up for yourself, but stick with it. The temporary discomfort will end up shielding you from far more distress down the line. At the end of the day, if people take issue with you prioritizing your personal peace, they can't be trusted to treat you well or act in your best interest. Among queer folks, we have a wide array of experience navigating the rejection of our true identities within our biological families.

"The more my dad lashed out, the further away I tried to get," says Jamal, who was raised in the South by parents who are fully committed to the gender binary and heteronormativity. "I had to do my own thing, which ultimately became distance. I've let that distance remain because I can't be around him knowing he's always going to preach at me or yell at me."

"My mother is very supportive, but that has taken many years and a lot of work on our relationship," says Lashan, a first-gen kid of Afro-Colombian descent. "My family is a lot more understanding of binary trans partly because Spanish is a binary language, and Colombia had a major trans rights movement in the nineties."

For some people, cutting off one of their parents was the best decision for them. Other nonbinary and trans folks I spoke to conveyed that they'd found space to work through their family's resistance to gender variance. These may not be your experiences, but if you've struggled with or lost family over bigotry, know that you are not alone. The tradition of absorbing nonbiological kin into family units is a longstanding practice in vulnerable communities. Marked by values of interdependence and mutual helpfulness, the communal strength of voluntary families has supported the collective survival of folks during periods of extreme abuse. Queer folks have intuitively adopted this survival skill of developing intentional families. You can, like so many others, develop deep connections with chosen family who will support you and allow you to fully show up authentically.

CREATING SAFER SPACES

Focus on approachable and joyful ways to work on dismantling negative internalized beliefs about your identity. A sense of safety and security is fundamental for healing spaces. Colonization interrupted BIPOC's connections to themselves by disrupting their communities, so finding affirming spaces where BIPOC folks can come together and take a break from white-centered spaces is crucial. People recovering from racial trauma and heterosexist discrimination need time and space to recover from the abuse they've been subjected to. It is cruel to ask for the wounded to prioritize the feelings of the unharmed as they seek out care. Give yourself permission to conserve your emotional energy and set boundaries with people who aren't willing to understand how you have been harmed.

There is a growing number of safe and welcoming places where people of color, queer folks, and gender-nonconforming individuals create community. If you find yourself in a space where you aren't encouraged to speak the truth when you observe hateful or exclusionary behavior, please keep it moving. You deserve better, and you can do better. Instead of throwing pearls before swine and wasting emotional energy on people who have no interest in seeing your humanity, please use that energy to locate communities that celebrate and validate you. These communities may not be in your immediate vicinity, but location is no longer a barrier to finding your village, thanks to the internet. Your people won't necessarily look like you or emote or love the way you do. Your chosen or found family is simply a collection of imperfect but genuine people who vibe with you, accept you, and are invested in your well-being.

"As a whole, people are shit, but I love my people," says Jamal, who found family in loving exes and childhood friends, but ultimately relocated to a larger city to connect with a sizable LGBTQIA+ community. "Where family has failed me, I have found good people who are as close to blood as they could get, and they're all shapes, all sizes, all colors. It just goes to show that it doesn't matter what someone looks like or where they've been or where they're from; you gotta give people a chance so you can find your real people.

"When the world was on fire around us, they knew I had them. I've always felt like that's what I needed to know, like *OK, no matter what, you're gonna be there, and I have somewhere to go.*"

The more your self-acceptance grows, the greater your tolerance for others' imperfections may become. Understanding that no one is perfect, ourselves included, is helpful as we build new relationships. That said, deep self-acceptance and self-love will not allow ongoing engagement with harmful people. Once you understand your value, accepting unwarranted abuse and neglect will no longer make logical sense to you.

If you have trouble finding an intersectional and inclusive space, consider creating one of your own. There is a pattern of homophobia and transphobia in many communities of color. Rather than going with the flow in spaces where gay folks are forced to play down their queerness and trans people are treated with hostility, confront the community's exclusionary behavior. If people aren't trying to get it together, create your own space.

It isn't necessary to completely segregate yourself from white folks, but taking time to exist in BIPOC-centered spaces is healthy. Intersectionality is beautiful. Spending time with safer white folks can be uplifting if they celebrate your whole self and are part of your blood or chosen family, but the value of connecting in safe BIPOC spaces can't be replaced by white loved ones. After years of being trained to play down all parts of yourself that aren't celebrated or valued by the dominant culture, being in the presence of your affinity group is the best way to learn that it's safe to fully be yourself.

If a trusted white person in your life questions this need or is offended by it, seriously think about whether you want to invest energy in explaining your experience to them. I have spent more time than I'd care to admit attempting to explain to insincere people that carving out safe spaces for POC is not "reverse racism." Remember, and feel free to remind white allies, that you don't need permission from anyone to pursue self-care. Invite them to spend less time policing POC behavior and more time investigating long-standing systems of oppression and their impact. People who can effortlessly be surrounded by members of their cultural group, awash in affirming images of themselves on a daily basis, have no business telling people who don't have that privilege how to go about creating safe spaces. It is rude and a blatant microaggression to even ask for "justification" for building community. Google is not broken. Libraries have not vanished from the face of the earth. If they would honestly like to learn why demanding assimilation and having no interest in dismantling systems of oppression is problematic, they are free to start educating themselves without asking for emotional labor from the BIPOC folks in their lives who are already plenty tired from fighting systems of oppression every day.

Remember that it isn't your job to educate people. You have every right to prioritize your own well-being and refuse to expend emotional energy. If you feel like you have the will and strength to fight for space in a way that will benefit the people who come after you, then do it. If you feel like you'd rather focus on finding a place where you'll be safe and free to fully express the truth of your being, then do that. Your life, existence, and joy, in so many ways, is a form of resistance in itself. When you choose where to spend your time, money, and attention, you are voting for what you want to see more or less of in the world. When you withdraw your membership from a problematic group or organization, you are protesting. You don't have to march if you don't want to march. Opting not to engage with problematic groups or organizations is a powerful form of protest in itself.

A common criticism that I hear from members of the dominant culture is that if recipients of abuse or marginalized folks want change, we should be willing to educate people on why we expect to be treated as equal beings. The onus to educate others is not on us, no matter what arguments you hear. On the contrary, it is obscene to place the onus to educate others on the recipients of abuse. It is not your responsibility to teach people to respect you. Holding identities that are not seen as valuable by the dominant culture does not obligate you to spend your lifetime attempting to convince others of your value. Your unique identities are not the trouble. Bigotry is the problem. Individuals upholding systems of oppression are the ones who need to get cracking on learning how to be decent human beings. Would you ever consider asking a battered spouse to stay in the home until they'd managed to convince their abuser that they were suffering? Would you think that advice was helpful, loving, or justifiable on any level if you heard it? Obviously, the battered spouse needs to prioritize their well-being, escape the dangerous environment, and seek safety. In many cases, the abuser is likely suffering and has issues of their own, but that is not the responsibility of the survivor of the abuse.

The very framing of inclusion through a white lens tends to be problematic, as a nice-to-have self-improvement project. The tendency to center white feelings in discussions of racial trauma is one of many reasons why the very presence of white folks in spaces that are meant to be safe for BIPOC rarely end up being restorative. White feelings are not of greater importance than QTBIPOC lives. White feelings are not more important than QTBIPOC feelings. White people who come into designated "safer" spaces for marginalized folks and focus on their relatively minor discomfort of having to confront the ways in which white supremacy delusion has given them an unearned leg up is 101-level foolishness we don't have to make room for. There are plenty of people who have been called to do Anti-Bigotry 101 work with folks. We don't have to take that on. This is not our problem to fix. Asking the survivors of abuse to captain personal improvement projects for members of the dominant culture adds to the chronic stress that already compromises our well-being.

Chronically expecting free labor, emotional or otherwise, is colonizer trash if I've ever seen it. Discrimination hurts everyone. Racism, heterosexism, and transphobia stop people from living full lives and being free to show up in their wholeness to share their gifts with the world. White folks who don't grasp this are stuck in the belief that their participation in the fight for the liberation of all people is benevolent or generous. The assumption that POC love nothing more than being supporting characters to the dominant white narrative, having no storylines of our own, has been baked into the consciousness of many by film and television for years. If you think about how many magical Negro, Native American, or wise Asian mentor tropes you've watched in movies over the years, it's easy to understand why so many white folks have been brainwashed into believing that POC exist to support their growth and evolution. The utter failure to comprehend that gaining respect and validation from white folks is not a ubiquitous goal for folks of color is exhausting. Feel free to opt out and give dominant culture folks in your life the room to take responsibility for doing the work to liberate themselves from white supremacy delusion without draining your emotional energy. You don't have to dedicate your precious time to attempting to get faux allies to understand that while they are clearly the center of their universe, they are not the center of yours. You do not have to spend every minute of every day (while the oppressor and friends are out living it up) proving that things need to change. That is not your responsibility. Spending time in consciously built communities gives you a chance to celebrate your uniqueness in a way that isn't possible under the white gaze. Maybe one day this won't be true, but presently, it is what it is.

PERMISSION GRANTED

Learning to be kind to yourself, nurture yourself, and love yourself in a world that is begrudging with affection is a journey. Developing an embodied practice of self-love can take a variety of forms. Here are some ways you can shower yourself in affection:

- Allow yourself quiet time daily.

- Create a list of healers you'd like to work with. Celebrate accomplishments and treat yourself, as often as you see fit, by reaching out to these folks.

- Say no to everything that doesn't light you up. You don't have to sit through movies you don't want to see. You don't have to endure social gatherings that make you feel drained.

- Offer yourself kindness when you are having a difficult day and allow room to sit with your feelings.

- Indulge your creative spirit without judgment or expectations. Write poetry in private, paint, sketch, trace, color, or draw mandalas. There is no wrong way to express your creativity. When you are expressing your creativity as a way to generate joy, don't seek outside input on what you create.

- Limit your contact with people who don't build you up.

- Take care not to fall into the comparison trap with others online. Remember that there is no competition here. You are unique, and you don't need to run your life according to anyone else's timeline.

After you go through these ideas and add a couple of your own to your journal, pick a few practices that you are pretty confident will be uplifting. Skip anything that feels underwhelming. Trust your gut on this one. Don't overthink this. You can always circle back and make adjustments later. Stay in tune with how you feel when you care for yourself with one of these practices. You will be able to sense what is working for you if you take the time to listen to your body's feedback.

SELF-LOVE MADE SIMPLE

For many, it's easier to understand what kindness looks like when it's offered to others rather than yourself. Start thinking of yourself as a friend and try to treat yourself the way you would treat a friend in need of emotional support. If you were advising a friend on how to practice self-love in this moment, what would you say? Would you encourage them to ask what support would look like for them in this moment? How would you guide them toward fulfilling their true needs instead of turning to temporary coping tools? Now ask *yourself* these questions: How can I best show myself compassion right now? What is the most loving thing I can do for myself right now that will serve me both in the present and in the future?

After asking these questions, set a timer for five minutes and repeat the following statements, taking a deep breath after each:

I shower myself in kindness.
I trust my body.
I am valuable.
I am safe.
I am worthy of love.
I take care of myself.
I nurture myself.
I love myself.

8

HONORING YOUR ANCESTORS' WILDEST DREAMS

You carry all of us in your heart. We shall live in every breath you take. Every incantation you speak.
　　　　　—Tomi Adeyemi, *Children of Virtue and Vengeance*

t's no secret that colonization has influenced current Western values. Depending on how your ancestors got to this country, you may or may not have a clear idea of who they were. All some of us have are vague stories of who they might have been. Being raised in the South, I didn't even get an accurate version of what they may have lived through. In the public school setting, I was told on countless occasions from kindergarten onward that slavery really wasn't that bad, and the abusive image of plantation owners was "northern propaganda." As an adult with free access to information, as things slowly but surely improve, and with revisionist history being challenged by people who speak truth to power, I'm able to at least build a structure in my mind for what my ancestors' lives might have been.

The truth is the transatlantic slave trade was a vicious crime against humanity, full of mind-boggling amounts of violence against children and adults alike. When I think about my ancestors and what they survived so I could live, I am overwhelmed with a sense of grief and love. When I meditate on the kind of life they dreamed of for their children and grandchildren, what always comes to me clearly is that they would want me to feel free. The fact that their definition of what freedom would look like can't possibly match what freedom means to me in a modern context doesn't matter. The dream was for the feeling of freedom, the sense of autonomy and control over one's own body, one's own destiny. Being free for me means feeling free to be myself; free to speak my truth, unshackled by the expectations of others; free to demand equal treatment; free to follow my dreams; free to live my life without harassment and abuse, surrounded by people who love and respect me; free to love who I want, when I want, and how I want.

I don't believe our ancestors survived countless insults to their humanity for us to settle for scraps of freedom. We honor our ancestors by claiming full liberation. When we buy into systems of oppression that elevate white beauty standards, we spit in the faces of our ancestors. When we deliberately try to erase and play down the parts of ourselves that are seen as Black, Indigenous, or native—and this applies to any racialized identity—we are trying to hide our ancestors' faces.

JOURNALING BREAK

Turn your attention inward and ask yourself these questions:

What do you imagine your ancestors wanted for you?

_____

_____

_____

How do you honor their memories with your life?

_____

_____

_____

How do you become a good ancestor (advocating for freedom of all)?

_____

_____

_____

Are you trying to hide your family's face?

_____

_____

_____

In your mind's eye, what does total freedom look like to you?

_____

_____

_____

Remember that not all ancestors are blood relatives. Chosen family extends the opportunity to be ancestors to childless folks as well. Our actions now, the way we guide the generations that follow us, will play a big role in how QTBIPOC can access peace and happiness. When you look back at your own experience, what vital information was held from you that you can now share freely? For example, one of the nonbinary folks I had the opportunity to interview shared their crystal-clear vision of how they will manage gender when they have children.

"I'm very much pro not disclosing the genitals of my children prior to birth," says Lashan, reflecting on their experience of gender reveals in their personal life and among the families they serve in public health. "I'm also pro not disclosing the genitals of my children to people outside of caregivers for my children. I want my children to have access to self-determination, allowing them to have whatever options without imposing gendered rules on them, letting them do what they want, and making sure they have a very concrete understanding of what gender diversity can look like from birth. That way, if my child identifies with the gender they would have been assigned at birth, then that understanding (not decision) is completely self-directed.

"I know some people are very much like, 'I'm going to raise my child as this gender because that's what they're being assigned and if they tell me they are different, then we'll switch it up.' I feel like that's kind of counterintuitive, and it treats being gender diverse as being abnormal or strange or something you have to work around. And that's not true; that's not helpful when it comes to creating the future we want to see and normalizing being gender diverse. Normalization doesn't look like 'We're going to assume you're this thing until you tell us otherwise.' That's not treating something like it's normal; that's treating it as an abnormality."

Imagine how life-changing it would have been to be told by an adult or caregiver early in life that gender nonconformity is a normal part of human diversity. How different would your experience of sexuality have been if your sex education would have included LGBTQIA+ folks? We have the privilege of serving as elders and future ancestors for found family and blood relatives. We have the power to normalize our identities for young folks by living as the most authentic versions of ourselves. The more you work on your decolonization and progress on your journey to radical self-love, the better equipped you are to become an ancestor who leaves love and liberation as part of their legacy.

ANCESTRAL LOVE

We all know about the intensity of the love parents have for their children. The way a parent's eyes light up when they look at their infant for the first time speaks to this intensity. It can be harder for us to imagine the depth of the love our ancestors have for us, because we haven't seen a firsthand demonstration of this type of familial love. Just think of the love parents have for their children, the admiration and love grandparents have for their grandchildren, and multiply that.

Honoring and connecting to ancestors is a longstanding tradition in many Indigenous communities of color, and is one of the oldest practices in human spirituality. Ancestors are believed to offer advice and guidance to the living. For example, they are perceived as deeply invested in the well-being and happiness of

living descendants in African traditional religions. It is generally
believed that ancestors maintain a connection and interest in the
well-being of their living relatives who are currently under the
influence of dominant culture. A lot of us no longer have a strong
connection to our extended families and may feel lost when it
comes to the concept of being intensely invested in the well-
being of other people in our bloodline, but at our core, humans
are communal and naturally interested in honoring their helpful
spirit when they feel safe and secure.

Immersing yourself in your ancestral story can have a healing
effect. An obstacle a lot of us confront is that our collective his-
tories have been suppressed. If you have undergone mainstream
schooling dispensed by the dominant culture, you likely haven't
ever been offered information about your ancestors through anything but a white lens. But our ancestors existed independent of
European influence for millennia. How much do you know about
the history of your ancestors prior to colonization?

Africa is the cradle of humanity. Clearly, African history does
not begin with colonization or the transatlantic slave trade. The
scientific and cultural achievements of Indigenous African cultures are ignored by design. Celebrating the accomplishments of
a culture you wish to diminish and see as inferior makes no logical sense. This is why you haven't heard about the continent's
path of development independent from European influence.

Likewise, Indigenous communities were living in the Ameri-
cas for over twenty thousand years prior to the Europeans' arrival
in the fifteenth century. The limited stories we are taught about
the Indigenous experience through a colonizer lens is severely
lacking. What have you ever been taught in a mainstream schooling setting about Indigenous life in America prior to the 1400s?

It isn't fair, but if you would like to be informed about your ancestors' experiences on this terrestrial plane, you have to make a deliberate effort to learn about their experience through your own research. You can't rely on the oppressor for accurate information. For the past several hundred years, the upholders of white supremacist culture have been convinced and are actively convincing others that Africa has no culture and no scientific or artistic legacies to speak of. This assertion is absolutely not based on reality. The cradle of civilization doesn't exactly sound like a place that should be disrespected and pitied for a lack of culture. Egypt was just one of many developed precolonial civilizations. We still marvel at the Egyptians' understanding of math, technology, and art, which were exhibited thousands of years before Rome came into existence. Read about your lineage. Ask family, friends, and virtual connections for book recommendations and develop a running decolonization recommended reading list. Another brilliant benefit of creating community with other POC is that you can access cultural information that the dominant culture has no interest in or deliberately suppresses because it challenges the oppressor's cultural narrative.

Think about the legacy you'd like to leave behind. What kind of ancestor do you want to be?

COMMUNICATING WITH YOUR ANCESTORS

Ancestor veneration: the practice of honoring one's deceased biological (and nonbiological) kin that respects the roles they play in the daily lives of the living

Ancestor veneration is a longstanding practice all over the world. If you don't have a connection to rituals that connect you to your ancestors, you can lean on your intuition to create practices that feel right for you. Starting your day with meditation and reflection at your altar is a powerful morning ritual.

Different cultures have various traditions for home altars, but setting up a basic one can be very simple. All you need to get started is a white cloth and a representation of each element (earth, water, air, fire). Start with an empty surface in a quiet part of your home. You can use some white fabric or a flat sheet as an altar cloth. Add a small plant to represent earth; a glass of water to represent water; incense, sage, or sweetgrass to represent air; and a small candle to represent fire. Your altar is a working space; it doesn't have to be perfect right out of the gate. It's meant to change over time. You'll continually add and remove offerings when it feels right for you. Light your candle to call your ancestors in. If you don't feel sure of what to say, here is a general call you might make to them:

Elevated ancestors, both known and unknown, I call out to you. I call on you to remember and honor you.

To all my elevated ancestors, both known and unknown, please feel the love I have in my heart for you. Surround me with your light, love, and power as I prepare for my day. Thank you for protecting and guiding me and keeping me aligned to my highest purpose. I love all my ancestors, known and unknown. I invite all benevolent ancestors, known and unknown, into my home. I give respect to the realm of the ancestors. Help me connect to my inner wisdom. I give praise to all who came before me. I give gratitude for all who have guided and loved me. I ask for continued guidance and protection from harm.

Treat your relationship with your ancestors as you do your relationships with the living. Don't simply show up to take. Bring known ancestors gifts they were drawn to in life, like their favorite foods or drinks. Place an offering on the altar and thank them for all the gifts they passed on to you.

ENJOY YOUR JOURNEY

This book is meant to be a tool, perhaps one of many, you can use on your way to self-acceptance and liberation. When you first start your decolonization process, you may feel overwhelmed and lost as to where to start. Don't feel rushed. This is a marathon, not a sprint. We've been surrounded by white-centered values for so long; decolonization is an ongoing process.

There are a growing number of resources out there made by people who want to support you on your journey. If you want more support, please reach out for help. My podcast, *Body Liberation for All*, was created to share ideas and resources for working toward body liberation. This is just one resource you can use to stay connected to your mission of practicing a high level of self-care and nurturing. I've compiled more resources on page 147.

My wish is for you to feel as free and as happy as possible every day of your life. I leave you with a list of reminders. Pick what hits and save it somewhere you'll see it often, like a screensaver or a note on your bathroom mirror.

- All bodies are good bodies.
- I am enough.
- I deserve all the sweet things in life.
- I don't settle for partial liberation.
- I am worthy.

- I am strong. I set boundaries to protect myself.
- I deserve self-care.
- I honor and satisfy my cravings.
- I trust my body.
- I trust myself.

I wish you peace, love, freedom, and happiness. You have permission to embrace joy and start living your life right now. Don't wait another day. This is your time.

ACKNOWLEDGMENTS

I am so grateful for the love and support I received from my community that made this book possible.

Thank you, Terry, for supporting my growth and liberation even when you didn't have a frame of reference to understand my experience.

Thank you, Rob and Papo, for always rooting for me and giving me space to be myself.

Thank you, Carmin, for your endless positivity and for validating that this message needed to be heard.

Thank you, Donnika, for giving me priceless feedback and encouragement to dream big and share my gifts with the world.

Thank you, Jesi Vega, for being a brilliant writing coach and giving me the confidence and direction I needed to pitch this book to BenBella.

Thank you, Vy, for giving clear feedback to make this book as strong a healing tool as possible for our community.

Thank you to the entire BenBella team for amplifying this message and being a delight to work with.

RECOMMENDED RESOURCES

Visit www.daliakinsey.com/resources for up-to-date suggestions.

Clothing

Binders—gc2b.co

Chest Binding Safely—Rachel Lisner, "Your Guide to Chest
Binding Properly and Safely," *Allure*, April 23, 2020,
https://www.allure.com/story/chest-binding-guide
-recommendations-tips.

Podcasts

Body Liberation for All, https://www.daliakinsey.com/bodylibpod

Yellow Glitter, https://yellowglitter.libsyn.com/

Books

The Body Is Not an Apology by Sonya Renee Taylor (Berrett-
Koehler, 2021)

Rainbow Reflections: Body Image Comics for Queer Men by Stephanie Gauvin, Phillip Joy, and Matthew Lee (Ad Astra Comix, 2019)

Wellness

GaneshSpace—ganeshspace.com
National Queer & Trans Therapists of Color Network—nqttcn.com
Point of Pride—pointofpride.org
Blackline (QTBIPOC helpline)—callblackline.com
Desi LGBTQ+ Helpline—deqh.org
Trans Lifeline (trans peer support)—translifeline.org
Sun Seed Community—sunseedcommunity.com

NOTES

INTRODUCTION: DECOLONIZING YOUR MIND

1. Christopher J. Pannucci and Edwin G. Wilkins, "Identifying and Avoiding Bias in Research," *Plastic Reconstructive Surgery* 126, no. 2 (2010): 619–625, doi:10.1097/PRS.0b013e3181de24bc.
2. "Registered Dietitian (RD) and Registered Dietitian Nutritionist (RDN) by Demographics," Commission on Dietetic Registration, accessed April 26, 2021, https://www.cdrnet.org/registry-statistics-new?id=1779&actionxm=By Demographics.
3. Alpana K. Gupta, Mausumi Bharadwaj, and Ravi Mehrotra, "Skin Cancer Concerns in People of Color: Risk Factors and Prevention," *Asian Pacific Journal of Cancer Prevention* 17, no. 12 (2016): 5257–5264, doi:10.22034/APJCP.2016.17.12.5257.
4. Xiao-Cheng Wu, Melody J. Eide, Jessica King, Mona Saraiya, Youjie Huang, Charles Wiggins, Jill S. Barnholtz-Sloan, et al., "Racial and Ethnic Variations in Incidence and Survival of Cutaneous Melanoma in the United States, 1999–2006," *Journal of the American Academy of Dermatology* 65, no. 5, supplement 1 (2011): S26–37, doi:10.1016/j.jaad.2011.05.034.
5. Chris Perez, "Education Company Under Fire for 'Racist' Nursing Textbook," *New York Post*, October 18, 2017, https://nypost.com/2017/10/18/education-company-under-fire-for-racist-nursing-textbook/.

CHAPTER 1: RESPECTING YOURSELF IN A HATEFUL WORLD

1. Sarah A. Tishkoff and Kenneth K. Kidd, "Implications of Biogeography of Human Populations for 'Race' and Medicine," *Nature Genetics* 36, no. 11 (supplement) (2004): S21–S27, doi:10.1038/ng1438.

2. Nina G. Jablonski, *Living Color: The Biological and Social Meaning of Skin Color* (Berkeley: University of California Press, 2012).

3. Angela Saini, *Superior: The Return of Race Science* (Boston: Beacon Press, 2019).

4. Charlotte R. Pennington, Derek Heim, Andrew R. Levy, and Derek T. Larkin, "Twenty Years of Stereotype Threat Research: A Review of Psychological Mediators," *PLOS One* 11, no. 1 (2016), https://doi.org/10.1371/journal.pone.0146487.

5. Arline T. Geronimus, Margaret Hicken, Danya Keene, and John Bound, "'Weathering' and Age Patterns of Allostatic Load Scores Among Blacks and Whites in the United States," *American Journal of Public Health* 96, no. 5 (2006), 826–833, doi:10.2105/AJPH.2004.060749.

6. Rolanda Lister, Wonder Drake, Baldwin Scott, and Cornelia Graves, "Black Maternal Mortality—The Elephant in the Room," *World Journal of Gynecology & Women's Health* 3, no. 1 (2019), doi:10.33552/wjgwh.2019.03.000555.

7. David Chae, Amani Nuru-Jeter, Nancy Adler, Gene Brody, Jue Lin, Elizabeth Blackburn, and Elissa Epel, "Discrimination, Racial Bias, and Telomere Length in African-American Men," *American Journal of Preventive Medicine* 46, no. 2 (2014), 103–111, doi:10.1016/j.amepre.2013.10.020.

8. Geronimus et al., "'Weathering' and Age Patterns."

9. Christian González-Rivera, Courtney Donnell, Adam Briones, and Sasha Werblin, "Funding the New Majority: Philanthropic Investment in Minority-Led Nonprofits," Greenlining Institute, Spring 2008, http://greenlining.org/wp-content/uploads/2013/02/FundingtheNewMajority.pdf; Paul Sullivan, "In Philanthropy, Race Is Still a Factor in Who Gets What, Study Shows," *New York Times*, May 1, 2020, accessed November 28, 2020, https://www.nytimes.com/2020/05/01/your-money/philanthropy-race.html.

10. Amy Bombay, Kim Matheson, and Hymie Anisman, "Intergenerational Trauma: Convergence of Multiple Processes Among First Nations Peoples in Canada," *International Journal of Indigenous Health* 5, no. 3 (2009): 6–47, https://doi.org/10.3138/ijih.v5i3.28987.

11. Robert T. Carter, Veronica E. Johnson, Katheryn Roberson, Silvia L. Mazzula, Katherine Kirkinis, and Sinead Sant-Barket, "Race-based Traumatic Stress, Racial Identity Statuses, and Psychological Functioning: An Exploratory Investigation," *Professional Psychology: Research and Practice* 48, no. 1 (2017): 30–37, https://doi.org/10.1037/pro0000116.

12. Ilan H. Meyer, "Prejudice, Social Stress, and Mental Health in Lesbian, Gay, and Bisexual Populations: Conceptual Issues and Research Evidence," *Psychological Bulletin* 129, no. 5 (2003): 674–697, doi:10.1037/0033-2909.129.5.674.

13. Stephen O. Murray and Will Roscoe, *Boy Wives and Female Husbands: Studies of African Homosexualities* (New York: Palgrave, 1998).

14. Karl Peltzer, Supa Pengpid, and Caryl James, "The Globalization of Whitening: Prevalence of Skin Lighteners (or Bleachers) Use and Its Social Correlates Among University Students in 26 Countries," *International Journal of Dermatology* 55, no. 2 (2016): 165–172, doi:10.1111/ijd.12860.
15. Matthew McKay and Patrick Fanning, *Self-Esteem: A Proven Program of Cognitive Techniques for Assessing, Improving and Maintaining Your Self-Esteem* (Oakland, CA: New Harbinger Publications, 2000).
16. Victoria M. O'Keefe, LaRicka R. Wingate, Ashley B. Cole, David W. Hollingsworth, and Raymond P. Tucker, "Seemingly Harmless Racial Communications Are Not So Harmless: Racial Microaggressions Lead to Suicidal Ideation by Way of Depression Symptoms," *Suicide and Life-Threatening Behavior* 45, no. 5 (2015): 567–576 doi:10.1111/sltb.12150.
17. Shiela Wise Rowe, *Healing Racial Trauma: The Road to Resilience* (Downers Grove, IL: InterVariety Press, 2020).

CHAPTER 2: ESCAPING THE DIET TRAP

1. Christy Harrison, *Anti-Diet: Reclaim Your Time, Money, Well-Being and Happiness Through Intuitive Eating* (New York: Little Brown Spark, 2019).
2. Sabrina Strings, *Fearing the Black Body* (New York: NYU Press, 2019).
3. Naomi Wolf, *The Beauty Myth: How Images of Beauty Are Used Against Women* (New York: Harper Perennial, 2002).
4. Letitia Anne Peplau, David A. Frederick, Curtis Yee, Natalya Maisel, Janet Lever, and Negin Ghavami, "Body Image Satisfaction in Heterosexual, Gay, and Lesbian Adults," *Archives of Sexual Behavior* 38, no. 5 (2009): 713–725, https://doi.org/10.1007/s10508-008-9378-1.
5. Matthew B. Feldman and Ilan H. Meyer, "Eating Disorders in Diverse Lesbian, Gay and Bisexual Populations," *International Journal of Eating Disorders* 40, no. 3 (2007): 218–226, doi:10.1002/eat.20360.
6. Elizabeth Diemer, Julia Grant, Melissa Munn-Chernoff, David Patterson, and Alexis Duncan, "Gender Identity, Sexual Orientation, and Eating-Related Pathology in a National Sample of College Students," *Journal of Adolescent Health* 57, no. 2 (2015):144–149, doi:10.1016/j.jadohealth.2015.03.003.
7. "The U.S. Weight Loss & Diet Control Market," Research and Markets, March 2021, https://www.researchandmarkets.com/reports/5313560/the-u-s-weight-loss-and-diet-control-market.
8. Kevin D. Hall and Scott Kahan, "Maintenance of Lost Weight and Long-Term Management of Obesity," *Medical Clinics of North America* 102, no. 1 (2018): 183–197, doi:10.1016/j.mcna.2017.08.012.

9. Sylvia Tara, *The Secret Life of Fat: The Science Behind the Body's Least Understood Organ and What It Means for You* (New York: W. W. Norton, 2017).

10. Traci Mann, Janet Tomiyama, and Andrew Ward, "Promoting Public Health in the Context of the 'Obesity Epidemic': False Starts and Promising New Directions," *Perspectives on Psychological Science* 10, no. 6 (2015): 706–710, doi:10.1177/1745691615586401.

CHAPTER 3: EATING AS SELF-CARE

1. Elizabeth A. Pascoe and Laura Smart Richman, "Perceived Discrimination and Health: A Meta-Analytic Review," *Psychological Bulletin* 135, no. 4 (2009): 531–554, doi:10.1037/a0016059.

2. Russell B. Toomey and Karla Anhalt, "Mindfulness as a Coping Strategy for Bias-Based School Victimization among Latina/o Sexual Minority Youth," *Psychology of Sexual Orientation and Gender Diversity* 3, no. 4 (2016): 432–441, doi:10.1037/sgd0000192.

3. Theodoros Angelopoulos, Alexander Kokkinos, Christos Liaskos, Nicholas Tentolouris, Kleopatra Alexiadou, Alexander Dimitri Miras, Lordanis Mourouzis, et al., "The Effect of Slow Spaced Eating on Hunger and Satiety in Overweight and Obese Patients with Type 2 Diabetes Mellitus," *BMJ Open Diabetes Research and Care* 2, no. 1 (2014): e000013, doi:10.1136/bmjdrc-2013-000013.

CHAPTER 5: LIBERATING YOURSELF
FROM BODY SHAME

1. Marie Kondo, *The Life-Changing Magic of Tidying Up: The Japanese Art of Decluttering and Organizing* (Berkeley, CA: Ten Speed Press, 2014).

2. Bessel van der Kolk, *The Body Keeps the Score: Brain, Mind, and Body in the Healing of Trauma* (New York: Penguin Books, 2015).

INDEX

ABOUT THE AUTHOR

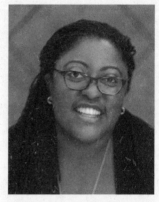

Photo by Jerrina Montgomery

Dalia Kinsey is a registered dietitian, decolonized wellness coach, and host of the *Body Liberation for All* podcast. Dalia works to make wellness accessible to all through inclusive wellness programs, along with public speaking engagements and workshops for providers who would like to create safer spaces for marginalized folks.

Visit www.DaliaKinsey.com to learn more about Dalia's work.